Health Disclaimer

This manual presents information based upon the research and personal experiences of the author. It is not intended to be a substitute for a professional consultation with a physician or other healthcare provider. Neither the publisher not the authors can be held responsible for any adverse effects or consequences resulting from the use of any of the information in this manual. They cannot be held responsible for any errors or omissions in the manual. If you have a condition that requires medical advice, the publisher and author urge you to consult a competent healthcare professional. Please consult your physician or other healthcare professionals for all personal health problems, and also before starting a new physical fitness program. No health information in this manual should be used to diagnose, treat, cure or prevent any medical condition. Anyone who has been inactive for several years and is over 35 years of age, should consider seeing a physician before any exercise program. Any application of the recommendations set forth in the following pages is at the reader's discretion and sole risk.

© 2006 by Paul Zaichik

Photography by Matthew Hanlon (Pages 27-146)

I would like to extend special thanks to everyone who helped make this project successful. Especially to Matthew Hanlon for his genius photography work. With his dedication and expertise he was able to capture the essence of The Gravity Advantage Max Program. Matt's other work can be seen at www.MatthewHanlon.com

ISBN # 1-933570-88-1

TABLE OF CONTENTS

ABOUT THE AUTHOR

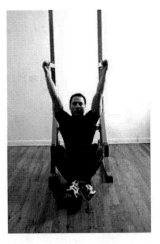

Paul Zaichik is the founder of The Elastic Steel Method of Athletic Conditioning, The Gravity Advantage & The Gravity Advantage MAX Programs.

Paul's childhood dream was to practice martial arts. In 1990, after years of playing other sports, he had enrolled in Martial Arts dojo. Since then every day's practice had become his passion.

A few years later Paul had taken up the Graduate and Undergraduate study of Exercise Science and Nutrition. Over the years, he had witnessed hundreds of instructors teach classes. By that time Paul had experimented with dozens of theories of exercise conditioning.

After years of practice, trial and error, the Elastic Steel Method of Athletic Conditioning & The Gravity Advantage Programs were born. Thousand of students have benefited greatly from this Method.

ABOUT THE GAM PROGRAM

Elastic Steel Method of Athletic Conditioning was inspired by a number of great systems of Arts. The Method draws upon Yoga, Pilates, Dance, Gymnastics, Track and Field and a variety of Martial Arts styles. Also, this method is greatly influenced by recent research in the area of Exercise Science.

Although this method has a strong orientation toward the fighting arts, it has been used successfully by a whole array of students. From people trying to tone up and lose weight, to high level athletes. From actors to everyday individuals recovering from injuries.

The focus of this program is on the development of total body strength. The approach taken is very unique. Only total body-weight lifting exercises are used. Maximum body-weight resistance training is applied to virtually every muscle group. Twelve exercises are required to cover all the muscle groups. Six of them target the upper body and six target the lower. Great emphasis is placed on the stabilization work of the midsection.

Many of the techniques taught in this program are unique and not widely known. This manual does more than just presents you with unique exercises. It also demonstrates sequences of progression that gently increase your skill and strength level, building up your body so that you are able to perform every one of the main techniques in this program.

The more exotic or unique a technique is, the longer sequence of progression it has.

Anyone who masters the twelve exercises in this manual will have a great looking, well balanced physique. So let's begin.

INTRODUCTION

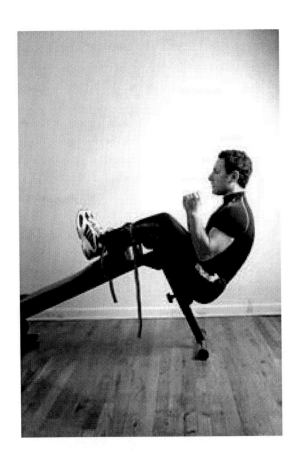

Since eternity, the human race has sought different ways to develop strength. When the struggle for survival was the only life that humans knew, one thing was certain: Strength was the leading factor that ensured survival. There were other factors; skills, cleverness, size of the group, weapons used, absence of disease, adequate supply of food and water. Still, above all was strength.

As humans evolved, they began to understand that strength can be improved through physical exercises. This meant that the weak could get stronger. This was a very attractive proposition. Having strength allowed people to protect or expand their territories, win wars, and of course survive.

Exercising using one's one body weight was one of the primary training techniques. A person's body weight is always with him. He never has to carry around any objects required for exercising. Gyms, resistance bands, the like were not available back in the day. Heavy items made out of rock, bone and metal were made available later on. Even these objects in most cases were expensive to make. Body weight exercises as well as the foot work drills were the training methods of choice.

Till this day, despite all the available machines the practice of using one's own body weight as resistance has survived. It is hard to meet someone in the civilized world who does not have a direct experience with body weight exercise, such as push ups. Military, as well as physical education classes, not to mention specialized physical arts, such as martial arts and dance, place great emphasis on body weight exercises. The reasons for this choice is usually the same. Body weight exercises are space economical. No or little equipment is required. Body weight exercises are generally accepted as safe.

When someone mentions body weight exercises, usually three moves come to mind. Pull ups, push ups, and dips. The very next thing that comes to mind, when this subject is brought up are squats, lunges, and sit ups . These are all great exercises, and anyone who does them regularly can get into great shape. Numerous variations of the above movements, such as limbs far apart or close together can add variety to these technique. Keeping this in mind it's important to understand that the above mentioned exercises, when taken together, lack two important components of the perfect exercise program.

Number one, they lack mechanical equilibrium and number two they don't reach the complete potential of strength development.

Anyone who knows a little bit of anatomy would know that standard push ups develop chest, front of the shoulder and triceps. Isometrically they also strengthen the front of midsection and legs. Dips strengthen front of the shoulders, triceps and mostly sternal part of the chest. Standard pull ups develop elbow flexors, latissimus dorsi, and teres major. Some effort is required on the part of the lower chest and posterior deltoid. All three exercises also work the movers and stabilizers of the scapula or the shoulder girdle.

As you can see, none of the three traditional body weight exercises have a counter exercise. A functional balancer, if you will. For example, push ups push forward, thus requiring an exercise that pulls back with the same force to provide harmony in the musculoskeletal apparatus. Pull ups exert a strong downward action pulling of the arms. Dips exert a strong downward pressing action. No balancing exercise is performed. Over time this hurts posture. In addition, it can lead to injuries and even culprits in health and well being. Gravity Advantage MAX just like Gravity Advantage is a program based on complete equilibrium. Every exercise is balanced. Moreover, not only are exercises paired action wise, they are also balanced in terms of resistance.

Complete use of body weight is the second issue. This program is designed to allow you to use your whole body weight on each lift. If you have mass, use it. Why lift a fraction of your body weight, when you can lift the whole weight, getting better results in the process. For example, standard push ups lifts roughly 2/3 of your body weight. Why settle for that, and not lift your whole body weight. developing your pushing power and the muscles associated with pressing movement.

Legs are often a neglected part of the body especially for males. But having well defined strong legs, goes far beyond looking great in shorts. It also makes you a better athlete. In sports where leg power is needed, whether for kicks, footwork, stances, jumps, or power transfer to the upper limb(s), having leg strength can make a world of difference.

This program teaches you how to develop the ultimate leg power and good looks using only your body weight as resistance. The second half of the manual teaches six exercises designed to develop the unparallel strength in the lower half of the body and the midsection.

Follow this program and let it change your life.

THE USE OF EQUIPMENT

Gravity Advantage Max program requires a few basic pieces of equipment. All six upper body exercises can be performed on two parallel (Dipping) bars. In upcoming chapters, as each exercise is introduced, substitution of the equipment may be suggested. Other props such as chairs, wall and high bar are incorporated to increase or decrease the level of difficulty.

The lower body exercises require the use of a bench. Flat bench or incline bench can be used. It's advised to use a padded bench. Sit up bench is ideal since it has the padding under the knees. However, if a regular wooden bench is used, some form of padding such as a matt would be recommended.

Some of the lower body exercises require the stabilization of the lower legs. This can be accomplished with the use of a belt or a strap. In many cases a partner can hold the legs in place. Exact spotting and application will be described in upcoming chapters.

Finally the chairs should be kept on hand. They will prove to be a useful tool for some of the progression techniques. Most equipment described above can be easily purchased in a local sports store. Parks and play grounds usually provide plenty of bars, both dipping and chinning. Weight lifting belt, although a comfortable choice, can be replaced by the straps. These can be found anywhere and are usually inexpensive. At the same time we have developed a special strap designed specifically for Gravity Advantage Max program. Check GravityAdvantage.com for details.

A bench is a worthy investment for this program. Some sports stores sell it for as low as $40.00. If you choose to make your own bench, the cost can be significantly reduced.

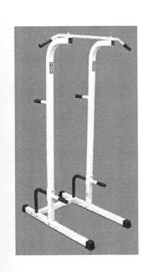

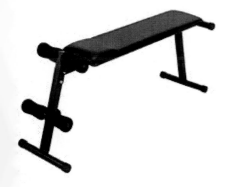

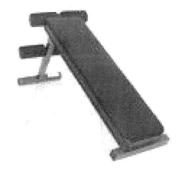

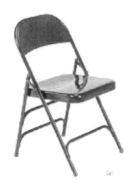

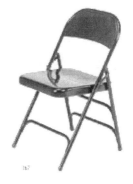

13

GETTING STARTED

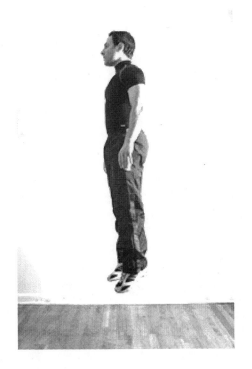

We are ready to begin. I strongly recommend that you spend some time on every part of the preparatory sequence before attempting the last exercise in the sequence. There are exceptions of course. If you can perform pull ups, there is no reason for you to abandon them and start the pull up sequence from the beginning. At the same time, if you have been successfully practicing the hyper extensions, there is no reason for you to abandon those in favor of superman extension, which are earlier in the sequence. On the other hand, if you have never worked on hyperextensions or superman extensions, then you should spend some time practicing the superman extension, prior to hyper extensions.

Remember the slower you go, the further you will get. It's important to understand that you are developing strength even if you don't do the most advanced exercises. Test yourself and see what level you are in every sequence, chances are you won't be on the same level across the board.

You may be able to do pull ups and dips, but happen to be a complete beginner when it comes to handstand presses. Treat each exercise as a separate entity. Do not allow the strength or weakness in one area to influence any other domain.

When you know what level you are starting out at, decide what equipment is required at the moment. There is no point in purchasing the pull up bar if you can't do any exercises that require it. Having it on hand can lead you to premature attempts at strength levels that you are not ready for. Wait until you are completely ready then make the celebrated purchase of the needed equipment.

The exercises in this program are arranged in a specific sequence. For the majority of athletes this is the most practical arrangement. Everyone is an individual however, and what works for most people may not work for you. The upper body sequence starts with the most difficult and unfamiliar exercises and ends with the most familiar techniques. Opposite pushing and pulling movement are usually varied for best results.

Unlike the upper body, the lower body routine provides the muscle isolation exercises. (Upper body isolation exercises are found in my other book "The Gravity Advantage" which you can purchase at www.GravityAdvantage.com.) For this reason the compound exercises such as one leg lunge and air lunge are placed in the beginning of the sequence. If, however, you master those two exercises quickly, placing them at the end of the six exercise routine can be an option.

If you do decide to move the lower body exercises around, it is preferred that you keep the posterior chain exercises, such as dragon curl, ahead of the anterior chain exercises, such as L-Extension. Most people's posterior chain is usually weaker than the anterior chain. At the same time, it is generally accepted that it is safer to train the back prior to training the front.

A few words of advice about the routine split. I've found that this program works best if it is split into the lower body and the upper body days. It is practically impossible and not very prudent to perform all twelve exercises in one day. It is best to have 3 spaced upper body days and 3 spaced lower body days.

Your midsection will be worked as a stabilizer on both days. If you choose to add some additional core exercises then you must decide which day you would like to do them. Some students like to add the midsection work outs to the upper body days, and some to the lower. Whatever your choice is, it is best to have the core routine at the end of the work out. If you choose to train your core at the start of the work out, it may interfere with later exercises, since the stability of the midsection muscles is required for other techniques.

Try to separate the lower and upper body days. For example have one type of work out on Monday, Wednesday, Friday and the other on Tuesday, Thursday, Saturday. Leave one day for rest. Three day training is usually optimum for each muscle group, for these type of techniques.

If you start to feel sore at first, then two days a weak instead of three may be the solution. Decreasing the number or sets may be another way to go. Remember, do not over train. Training to failure is not recommended either. Unless you can only perform only a few repetitions of the exercise, stop one or two reps prior to reaching your maximum number of repetitions.

Only every few weeks when you test yourself, go all out. Other than that, stay away from over exertion.
Sometimes you may hit a plateau. This means that you can't increase the number of repetitions no matter how hard you try. Very often taking a week or a few days off can help the progress. Sometimes it is best to keep practicing other exercises while taking time off from the one that has hit a plateau.

Remember to warm up prior to every workout session. It's a fact that not everyone requires the same warm up. With practice you will be able to fine-tune the best way to get yourself ready for the work out. Here are the general recommendations.

Start your work out with joint rotations. These are simply circles performed with each joint. As simple as these movements may seem, they are very important for safe and effective work out. Here is the order.

- Wrist circles
- Elbow circles
- Shoulder circles
- Head circles
- Torso rotation
- Hip circles
- Knee circles
- Ankle circles

It is a good idea to cool down in the reverse order of the warm up. Slowly, while taking full deep breaths perform the same exercises you have used as you warm up. (Push ups, squats, etc.)

Following joint rotations, a light aerobic warm up is recommended. Jogging in place, jump rope, or a few minutes of jogging is a very common warm up activity. Following the aerobic warm up, specific warm up is recommended. If this is your upper body day, do 2 sets of 10 push ups, followed by 2 sets of 10 horizontal pull ups. When using these exercise as a warm up sometimes it's best to shuffle the sets. Do a set of push ups, followed by horizontal pull ups, followed by the push ups and then the horizontal pull ups one more time.

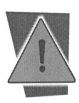

RESOURCE

Got a question about something that's been described so far?

Log on to **GravityAdvantage.com** and get answers from your fellow GAM practitioners!

If you are warming up for the lower body workout, squats are a great warm up technique. Do 2 sets of 10 –20 squats. Followed by 2 sets of 10 lunges. Some techniques require specific warm ups and those are listed individually in the chapters preceding each of the 12 exercises.

Stretching prior to strength workout is a matter of individual preference. Scientific literature is conflicting when it comes to this issue. Many experts believe that a thorough joint rotation warm up, few minutes of aerobics and a few sets of warm up exercises such as push ups or squats is all you need for a good strength performance.

Start a cool down with a few minutes of relaxed aerobic exercises. Slowing down the pace gently. Meaning if you decide to jog in place for 3 minutes, the first minute is most vigorous, decreasing pace with every passing minute.

Following the aerobic cool down, do the joint rotations. Slowly perform the circles using the full range of motion that the joints allow. At this point you may spend time on relaxed stretches. A stretching routine is provided at the end of the book.

JOINT WARM UP

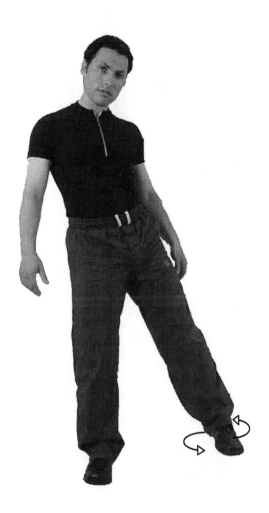

Position: *Wrist circles*

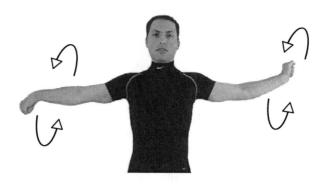

- **Action:** Circle your wrists 10-15 times in each direction.
- **Key points:** Perform the exercise slowly focusing on the movement.
- **Purpose:** To lubricate the writs joint, and warm up the fore-arm.

Position: *Elbow circles*

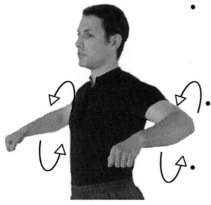

- **Action:** Perform 10-15 elbow circles in each direction. Imagine that you are hitting two speed bags with your hands, while your elbows stay pointed at the speed bags.
- **Key points:** Keep your flexing and extending your elbows, as you simultaneously rotate (not circle) your shoulder joints.
- **Purpose:** To lubricate the elbow and the shoulder joints. To warm up the upper arm muscles as well as shoulders.

Position: *Arm/shoulder circles*

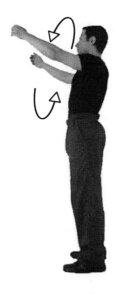

- **Action:** Perform 10-15 arms circles in each direction. Start with smaller amplitude and increase the diameter, with each consecutive repetition.
- **Key points:** Perform the movement in a controlled, continuous manner.
- **Purpose:** To lubricate the joints of the shoulder and the shoulder girdle. To warm up the muscles of the shoulder and the upper back.

Position: *Head circles*

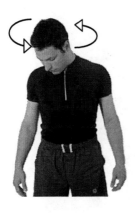 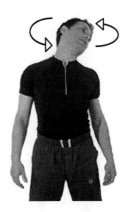

- **Action:** Perform 10-15 head circles in each direction.
- **Key points:** Perform the movements in controlled, continuous manner.
- **Purpose:** To lubricate the joints of the cervical spine. To warm up the muscles of the neck.

Position: *Torso rotation*

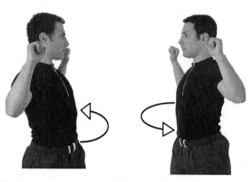

- **Action:** Rotate your trunk side to side.
- **Key points:** Keep the spine neutral.
- **Purpose:** To lubricate the joints of the spine. To warm up the muscles of the mid-section.

Position: *Hip circles*

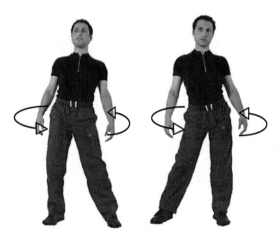

- **Action:** Perform 10-15 hip circles in each direction.
- **Key points:** Keep the spine neutral.
- **Purpose:** To lubricate the hip joint. To warm up the muscles responsible for the movement of the joint.

Position: *Knee circles*

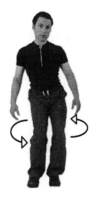 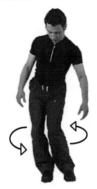

- **Action:** perform 10-15 knee circles in each direction.
- **Key points:** Stay within the normal range of movement.
- **Purpose:** To lubricate the knee joint.

Position: *Ankle circles*

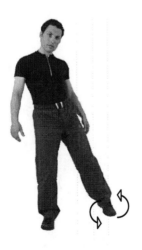 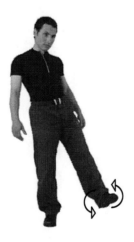

- **Action:** Circumduct your foot 10-15 times in each direction.
- **Key points:** Stay within the normal range of movement.
- **Purpose:** To lubricate the foot and ankle joints. To warm up the muscles responsible for the movement of those joints.

BODY PRESS

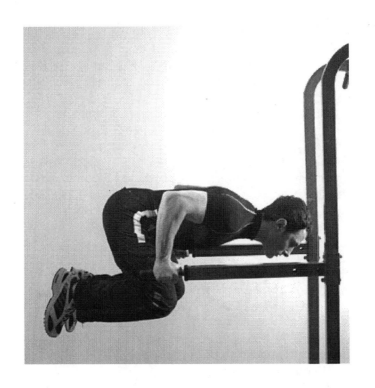

Body press is a body weight bench press, at least on some level. This exercise allows you to practice forward pushing movement with maximum body weight resistance. When you perform the regular push ups, depending on your body mass distribution and push up variation, you push roughly 70-75 % of your body weight. With the body press you increase the load. It is much more than that however. The struggle to maintain leverage and stability adds an additional benefit. To understand this, think of yourself doing push ups. How many can you do? Now imagine yourself practicing the same exercise with hands on the stability ball. What about each hand on a separate stability ball?

Will you be able to perform the same number of push ups as you have, with hands firmly on the floor? Probably not. You will most likely perform less. What changed? You are still lifting the same weight. The difference is in the muscle effort. Instead of only focusing on lifting your body, the focus is also on stabilization. Your muscles must do more work. A lot more work. Thus they fatigue faster.

As you can already guess, the same happens with body press. Your muscles struggle to maintain your body in horizontal position. Between that and fighting the resistance of your body, the exercise becomes very difficult.

This is a good concept, from both athletic point of view and muscle building point of view. When you are trying to build muscle tissue, there is no discrimination. Work is work. Struggling to maintain stability or struggling to lift the weight, both of those make the muscles bigger and stronger. A combination of those two factors is much better than either one.

From the point of view of an athlete, steadiness is just as important as strength. Any sport or athletic activity is multi directional. Talking about pushing movement think of a line backer or a power lifter. Line backers who push the other line man, must not only press, but stabilize their limbs, for their opponent will never stay still.

Having to push a moving target requires a lot more effort than pushing a stationary one. A power lifter who bench presses is up for a lot less surprises than a line man. Still the barbell is free to fall in any direction. Thus a bench press must stabilize the bar not only lift it.

Anyone familiar with strength training would know that a forward press on a machine or a bench press using the Smith machine is not the same as a free weight press. You can always press more weight when it is stabilized. The less leverage, the harder the exercise. In the case of the parallel press, leverage is part of the challenge.

The shoulder is the hardest worker when it comes to the body press. In order to be able to maintain a parallel position, the shoulder must be relatively well trained. It doesn't matter how much you can push, if your shoulder can hold the position, you won't be able to perform the body press. For this reason, most of the preparation exercises are focused on the shoulder strength. Beside the shoulder, your back extensors stabilize the lower body in parallel to the floor position. Super man is the exercise that strengthens the back muscles, which when activated extend your spine. This muscles groups also are the opponent muscles of the rectus abdominals or the six pack.

It is recommended that the quest for this skill begins with superman and push ups. Both exercises should be performed slowly, with control. Three sets of super man, should be intertwined with three sets of push ups. It's recommended not to train to exhaustion. Stop a few repetitions prior to complete failure.

While performing push ups, keep the elbows in. This will enhance the carry over to the body press. Three sets of 20-30 repetitions is good enough. Once that is achieved begin moving the hand further down, toward the hips. Depending on your wrist flexibility, you may want to point your fingers out or down. You can also use the fist, as demonstrated in the photos.

As for superman, begin with 3 sets of 20-30. Once you are able to perform 50 in one set, you are ready to move on.

Once you are able to place your hands directly under your hips and perform 10-15 non-stop push ups, it's time to move on to the pseudo planche and locust. This is the exercise that will ultimately prepare your shoulders as well as core stabilizers for the parallel press.

A key point to this exercise is to find the right hand position. You must place your hands so that they can support both your upper and your lower body. If the hands are too high up, they will not be useful in assisting in lifting the lower body. If, on the other hand, they are too low, you will not be able to lift the upper body.

A locust position is characterized by lifted legs in the prone position. Two facts need to be kept in mind in order to achieve this position. One is the use of the hands. Unless you are super strong and flexible, you will not be able to lift your lower body completely off the ground without the use of your arms. You must press with your hands into the floor and use the strength of the shoulders to lift the legs. Second is the breathing. As you breathe in, allow your abdominals to expand. As the diaphragm pushes down on your abdominal organs, they in turn push the abdominal wall out. Use the expansion of the abdominals and the lower body will be lifted higher than usual. Alternate lifting the lower and the upper body.

Once 15 repetitions are performed it is time to move on to the bars. In reality, two chairs can be served the same purpose as the dipping bars. If you choose to use the chair be prepared for greater challenge to your wrist.

I recommend accustoming yourself with the decline press prior to attempting the body press. The decline press is called that because the pressing movement is downward, regardless of the fact that the head level is above that of the legs. This exercise is an intermediate between the dips and the parallel press. Since your shoulders are already strengthened by the floor exercises, the feel for the suspended motion is need. Decline press helps you to experience that feel. Decline press also forces the thumb part of the wrist to take more pressure.

Notice that once you begin to practice the body press, the thumb part of the wrist must be prepared. This is due to the fact that the arms are not vertical as in push ups. The position of the arms in the body press is actually angular. This kind of constitution is required to keep the trunk horizontal. Decline press is not a necessity, only a supplement. You may want to try it, while you are preparing yourself with the floor exercises, so that once you mastered the floor exercises, you are more ready for the body press.

At this point all the muscles are ready, it becomes important to establish the straight arm position. The Parallel Open is the exercise that we need. Keeping your arms as straight as possible rotate forward from the dipping position to the parallel position. If you have prepared yourself with the floor exercise, parallel open should be achievable. Due to the novelty of the position it may take a few tries, but it can soon be mastered.

Once you are able to get into the parallel position, try to hold it for as long as comfortable. For many athletes this is the most difficult part. If you can come close to 20 seconds of holding the straight arm position, you may begin to practice the body press. Start by working on the negative movement. Come up to the straight arm body press position and come down to the bend arm position as slow as you can. Here number 3 is good to remember. Perform three sets of 3 negatives, 3 times a week. If after sometime you are not able to push yourself back up, increase the number of negative repetitions to 5, but stay with 3 sets.

Once you are able to perform one positive (concentric) contraction, stay with that one repetition for 3-6 sets. Space the sets out, and give yourself time to regain strength. With practice you will be able to decrease the rest intervals. Once you are able to perform two good repetitions, begin to perform 3 sets of 1 repetion and one set of 2. With time you should be able to perform 3 sets of one, followed by 3 sets of two. By the time you are able to perform 3 good repetitions, you can perform 3-6 sets of two.   The basic rule to follow here is not push the maximum, unless you are at only one repetition.

A good question to ask now is "How strong does this exercise really make you?" After having tried body press, I will leave you to answer this question for yourself. I have no doubt that you will know the answer.

In terms of warm up sequence for this exercise, I suggest the following.
- Two sets of ten push ups.
- Once set of pseudo planche push ups.
- 2-3 attempts of straight arm body press hold.

Following this, a warm up body press can be safely performed. And by the way, do not get lazy while working on the parallel open. While working on this technique remember to keep working on the pseudo planche and locust. You can stop practicing the pseudo planche and locus only after you have achieved that one perfect repetition of the body press. Great luck to you!

RESOURCE

Got a question about something that's been described so far? Log on to **GravityAdvantage.com** and get answers from your fellow GAM practitioners!

Superman

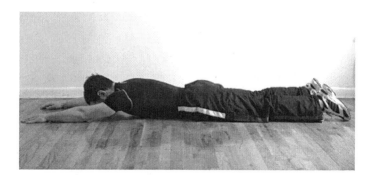

Pic. 1

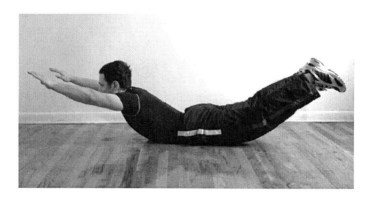

Pic. 2

- **Action:** Lie face down. Extend your arms and legs.(Pic.1) Lift your arms and legs up. (Pic. 2) Hold for 3 seconds and return to starting position.
- **Key points:** Keep the left and right limb at equal height.
- **Purpose:** To strengthen the lower back, in preparation for the parallel press.

Push Ups

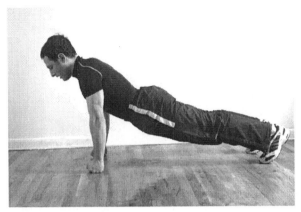

Pic. 1

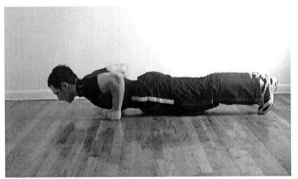

Pic. 2

- **Action:** Lie down on your stomach.(Pic.1) Place your hands under your rib cage. Press up (Pic.2) and return to the starting position.
- **Key points:** Keep the elbows close to the body.
- **Purpose:** To strengthen the upper body muscles necessary to perform the parallel press.

Pseudo Planche Push Ups

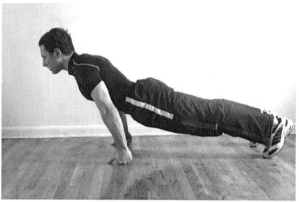

Pic. 1

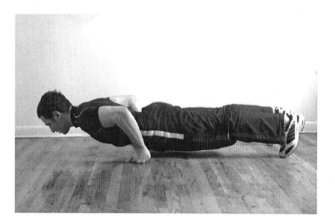

Pic. 2

- **Action:** Same as in previous exercise. Only the arms are under the hips.
- **Key points:** Try to keep the trunk in straight line.
- **Purpose:** To further strengthen the upper body in preparation
  for the parallel press.

Pseudo Planche and Locust

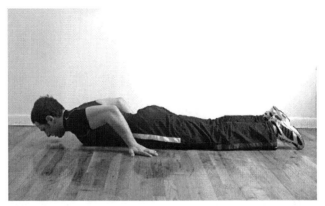

Pic. 1

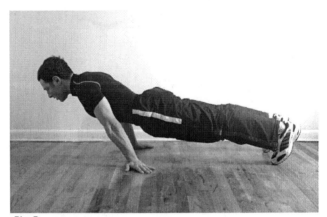

Pic. 2

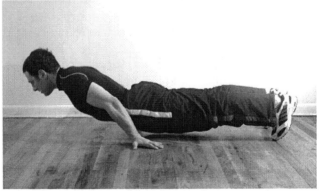

Pic. 3

Continued on next page...

Pseudo Planche and Locust

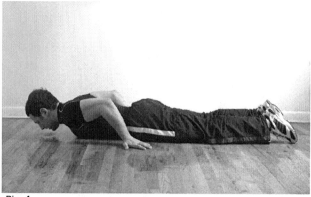

Pic. 4

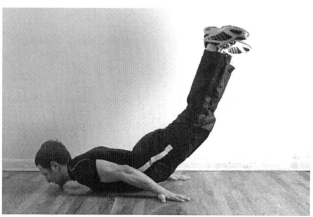

Pic. 5

- **Action:** Assume a push up position (Pic. 1). Place your hands under your hips/thighs. Press up, till the arms are extended as much as possible. (Pic. 2) Return to the floor.(Pic. 4) Without moving the hands, raise your legs off the ground. (Pic. 5) Return to the starting position.
- **Key points:** Aim to find the hand position, which you can hold without shifting.
- **Purpose:** To strengthen the shoulders and the core. To develop balance required to perform the body press.

Decline Press

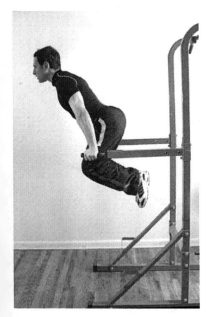
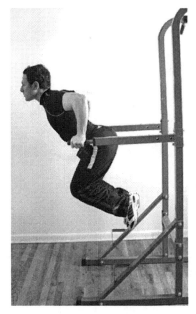

Pic. 1   Pic. 2

- **Action:** Assume a dipping position. Lean forward 45 degrees. (Pic. 1) Bend the elbows and lower your body. (Pic. 2) Press back up, to the starting position.
- **Key points:** Try to keep your head up and shoulder forward of the hands. (Shoulders are not directly above the hands, but slightly in front of the hands. Straight arms are not vertical, but rather at an angle.)
- **Purpose:** To strengthen the shoulders and the core. To get the feel for the shoulder as simultaneous mover and stabilizer. To strengthen the wrist.

Parallel Open

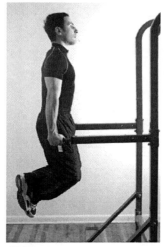

Pic. 1

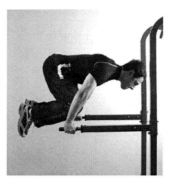

Pic. 2

- **Action:** Assume a dipping position. (Pic.1) Lean forward with your upper body. Lift your hips and tuck your knees (Pic. 2). Return to the starting position.
- **Key points:** Focus on lowering your chest down and forward.
- **Purpose:** To strengthen the shoulders and the core. To develop balance required to perform the parallel press. To strengthen the wrist.

Body Press

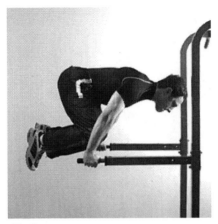

Pic. 1

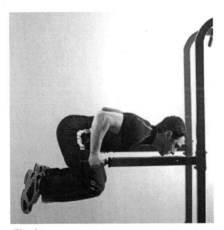

Pic. 1

- **Action:** Assume a straight arm body press position(Pic 1) .
- Lower your self as much as possible, by bending your arms (Pic. 2) . Return to the starting position.
- **Key points:** Focus on keeping the trunk parallel to the bars/ floor.
- **Purpose:** To strengthen the forward pushing muscles.

BODY ROW

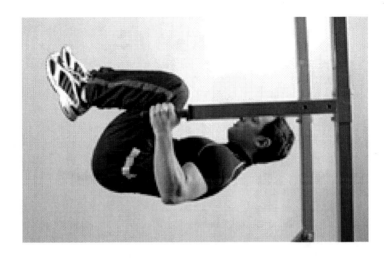

Body row is a complementary exercise to the body press. The former works the opponent muscles of the latter. While the body press works the anterior deltoid and pectorals major at the shoulder joint, the body rows works the teres major, latissimus dorsi and posterior deltoid. Core stabilizers are also balanced out by the two exercises. Body press recruits the rectus abdominals and to some degree oblique abdominals as stabilizers, while the body row relies on the extensors of the spine for trunk stabilization.

As a matter of fact, the two exercises even use the same exact resistance load– you own body weight.

It is not uncommon for body weight enthusiasts to excel in body rowing faster than body pressing. The reason is rather simple. Most athletes who use body weight exercises are accustomed to pull more weight than they can push. The most common pushing exercise is pull ups, while the most common pulling exercise is pull-ups. Although the two are not directly opposite of each other, push ups lift significantly less weight than do pull ups. Since pulling muscles are stronger the carry over is better, when another pulling exercise is attempted such as body rows. On top of that, the trunk stabilizers for the body rows are usually stronger and better developed that the one's used for the body press. In other words, the abdominals are usually trained more and harder than the back. So don't be surprised if you can bang out one or two repetitions on the first try. If that is the case with you, you may skip the progression sequence and go straight to body rows. For a method to increase the number of repetition take a look at page 32. Same method that applied to body press can be applied to this exercise.

The preparation sequence for the body row begins with the conditioning of the midsection and the pulling muscles. Reverse crunch is an exercise chosen to strengthen the abdominals. Three sets of this exercise are recommended to be performed 3 times a week, for a total of 9 sets a week. Start each set with as many repetitions as possible and build it up to 15-25 repetitions. Once this is achieved, the reverse crunch should be replaced with the pump. Work on achieving the same number of repetitions with this exercise. If done correctly both of these exercises will do more than just strengthen the core. They will also strengthen the back of the arms and back of the shoulder.

To strengthen the back of the arms and shoulders, legs must be lifted straight up and not in an arch over the body. If the legs are lifted up or away from the trunk, the arms would be forced to press against the floor for support. For our purpose, recruiting the arms is a desirable trait.

The first exercise in the pulling sequence is the horizontal pull up. This exercise is somewhat similar to the body row. The arm movement is partially the same, but the stability of the shoulders and the trunk is very different. Never the less horizontal pull up is a good pulling exercise, for this sequence. Start with 3 sets, 3 times a week. Work your way to 20-30 repletion for each set. Once 10 repetitions are achieved begin to incorporate Lizard into the sequence.

Lizard is recommended even for those who are masters when it comes to traditional pull ups. The reason being, that the pull ups allow the elbows to approach the sides of the body, but not pass it. To be successful with the body row, you must be able to pull your elbows back, way past your body. Rowing movement allows for this freedom of movement, pull ups do not. It is not uncommon for someone to be able to perform 10 pull ups, but not one Lizard. This is due to the fact that the muscles used for the hyper extension of the shoulder, are not trained while performing the pull ups. Same can be said for pull ups and body rows. The athletes expedited with pull ups, most likely would be able to start the body row, but not finish it. They are most likely to stop half way, when the bent elbows come close to the ribs. Practicing the Lizard helps to remedy this problem.

Lizard should usually follow the horizontal pull ups in the same sequence. As with the later exercise, practice three sets, 3 times a week.

Once the above four exercises are mastered. It's time to hit the bars. The remaining of the sequence will be demonstrated and described using the dipping bars. It the dipping bar is not available it is possible to use the high (Pull up bar). High bar will provide less stability and restrict full range of movement at the top of the exercises.

Parallel tuck hang is the exercise that strengthens the muscles required to hang in the horizontal position. Perform this exercise slowly. Once parallel to the floor, hold this position for few seconds and than descend.

Once you started working on the parallel tuck hang, it is not necessary to continue with abdominal exercises. The Lizard and the horizontal pull ups, should continue until at least one repetition of the body row is mastered.

If you are able to do pull-ups but can't do any body rows, there is an exercise which provides a transition. It's called the incline row. This exercise is a hybrid between the pull up and the body row. Practicing this exercise can get you closer to the goal of performing body rows.

Once you are able to hang parallel to the ground, you are ready for the next step. The negative or eccentric part of the movement. You may use the chair to get into the flexed arms position. Once there, hold it for as long as comfortable and descend slowly. Again remember the three. Three sets, three repetitions each per work out. Three work outs a week. Keep this up till you are able to do the concentric or positive movement. In other words until you are able to pull yourself up. At this point adopt the schedule described on page 32.

Here is the recommended warm up routine for this exercise:

- Horizontal pull ups 2 sets of 10-20.
- Flexed arms parallel hang 2-3 sets.

Begin the body rows! Shaped, powerful back awaits you.

Reverse Crunch

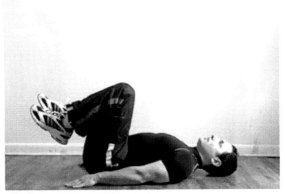

Pic. 1

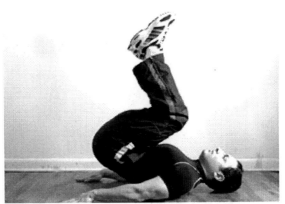

Pic. 2

- **Action:** Lie down on your back. Flex your hips and knees. (Pic. 1)
- Using the strength of the abdominals and the arms, lift the hips of the floor. (Pic. 2) Return to the starting position.
- **Key points:** Keep the head on the floor. Perform the movement slowly, do not use momentum to kick the legs up.
- **Purpose:** To strengthen the abdominals and back of the arms and shoulders, in preparation for the body row.

Horizontal Pull Ups

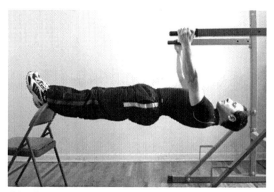

Pic. 1

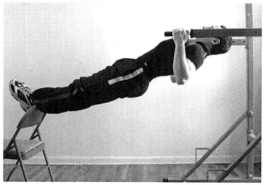

Pic. 2

- **Action:** Grip the dip bars with both hands. Place your feet, ankles or calves on the chair or another object of the similar height. (Pic.1) Pull your arms toward your chest or stomach. (Pic. 2) Return to the starting position.
- **Key points:** Keep the abdominals and glutes squeezed to protect the lower back.
- **Purpose:** To strengthen the pulling muscles in preparation for the body row.

Pump

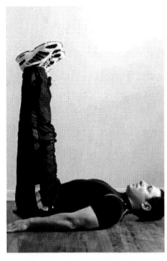

Pic. 1

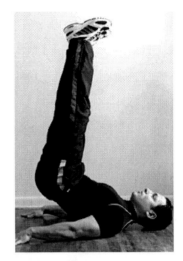

Pic. 2

- **Action:** Lie down on your back and place your arms by your side. Extend both legs directly toward the ceiling (Pic. 1). Using only the strength of the abdominals and the back of the arms, lift your hips up.(Pic.2) Return to the starting position.
- **Key points:** Do not use momentum to swing the legs up. Try to keep the legs as vertical as possible.
- **Purpose:** To strengthen the abdominals and the back of the arms/ shoulders in preparation for the body row.

RESOURCE

Got a question about something that's been described so far? Log on to **GravityAdvantage.com** and get answers from your fellow GAM practitioners!

Lizard

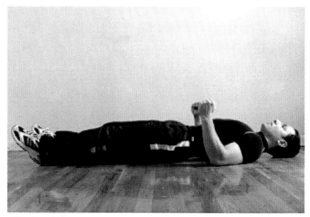

Pic. 1

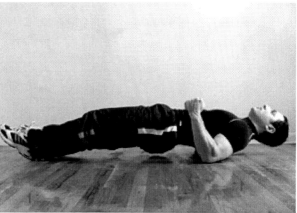

Pic. 2

- **Action:** Lie down flat on your back. Place your arms by your sides. Flex the elbows. (Pic. 1) Press down with your elbows and lift your hips. (Pic. 2) Hold for as long as comfortable and return to the starting position.
- **Key points:** Keep the shoulder blades squeezed together. Squeeze the glutes and abdominals to protect the lower back.
- **Purpose:** To strengthen the extensors of the shoulders.

Parallel Tuck Hang

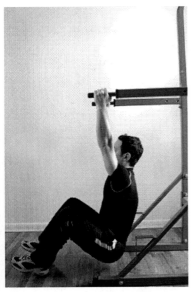

Pic. 1

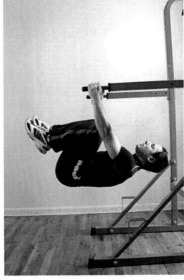

Pic. 2

- **Action:** Grip the bars with both arms. Lift your legs, so that your body is suspended. (Pic. 1) Lean back and lift your lower body up. (Pic. 2) Hold for as long as comfortable and return to the starting position.
- **Key points:** Allow the hands to remain over the abdominal area and not over the shoulders. Allow the arms to be slightly slanted and not completely vertical.
- **Purpose:** To get accustomed to the proper starting/ hanging position in preparation for the body row.

Pull Up to the Negative Body

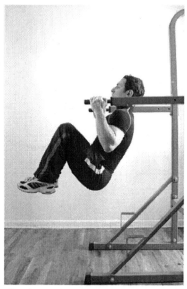

Pic. 1

- **Action:** Grip the bars with both hands. Pull yourself up to the starting position. (Pic. 1) Keeping your arms flexed, lean back. (Pic. 2) Hold this position for as long as possible and slowly extend your arms. (Pic.3)
- **Key points:** As your arms are extended, focus on keeping the trunk parallel to the floor.
- **Purpose:** To prepare for the full body row.

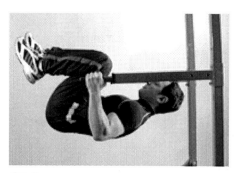

Pic. 2

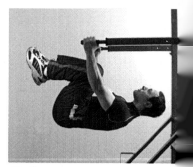

Pic. 3

Incline Row

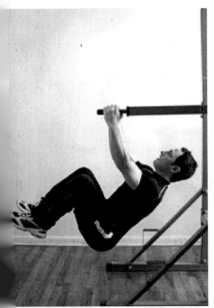 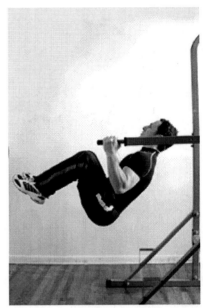

ic. 1   Pic. 2

- **Action**: Grip the bar with both hands. Lean back slightly so that the body is on the incline angle. (Pic. 1) Pull yourself up, maintaining the angle of he body. (Pic. 2) Return to the staring position.
- **Key points:** Keep your shoulder blades squeezed together.
- **Purpose:** To develop a transition from the pull ups to the body row.

Supine Grip Body Row

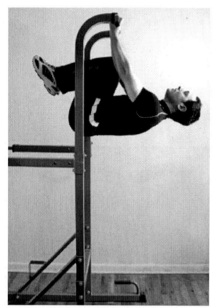 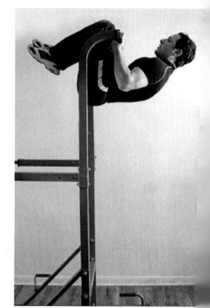

Pic. 1   Pic. 2

- **Action:** Assume a staring chin up position. Lift your lower body, till your trunk is vertical. (Pic. 1) Maintaining the position of the trunk, pull up. (Pic. 2) Return to the starting position.
- **Key points:** Hips may have to extend slightly to provide enough clearance for the bar.
- **Purpose:** To offer a variation of the body row.

Prone Grip Body Row

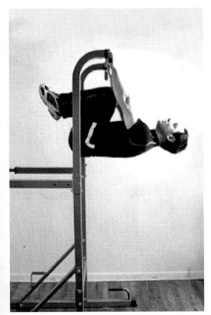 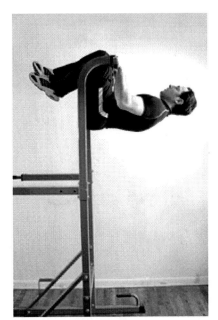

Pic. 1   Pic. 2

- **Action:** Assume a staring pull up position. Lift your lower body, till your trunk is vertical. (Pic. 1) Maintaining the position of the trunk, pull up. (Pic.2) Return to the starting position.
- **Key points:** Hips may have to extend slightly to provide enough clearance for the bar.
- **Purpose:** To offer a variation of the body row.

HANDSTAND PRESS

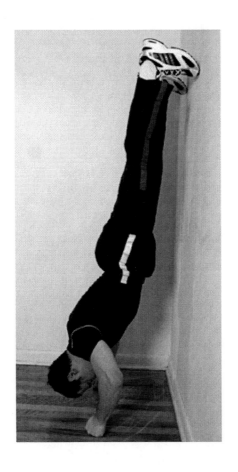

The hand stand press is one of the finest shoulder/ upper back development exercises. It is also an antagonist to the pull ups. As ancient saying goes "Don't be afraid of the man with huge arms, but rather of the man with big shoulders." Shoulders are positioned in the center of upper body movement. Most often a person with strong shoulders has other muscles developed as well. Hand stand press allows your whole body weight to be concentrated on your shoulders and triceps.

From my experience many people will find this exercise the most difficult one out of the 6 upper body exercises. There is a good reason for this. Shoulders are not large muscles. They are certainly smaller than latissimus dorsi, which is used in pull ups. At the same time, very few people have strong enough shoulders to press their own body weight.

The progression sequence is rather simple. Start with a familiar exercise, the push ups. From there keep slowly transferring the load away from the chest, and toward the shoulders, increase the resistance as you go along.

The sequence begins with incline push ups. Here we begin to concentrate on the upper chest and shoulders. To make this exercise effective, hold the bottom (bent arm) position for 3-5 seconds each time. Three sets, three times a week. Work your way up to 20-30 repetitions per set. Next try the same things with one leg lifted. Keep training till the same number or repetitions is achieved.

Once that is achieved begin to move the hands closer to the chair. Keep at it, till you are able perform three sets of 20-30 reps of the shoulder press push ups. At this point begin practicing the walk up. This goal of the walk up is to develop strength in the stabilizers need to perform the hand stand press. Start with your hands 3-4 feet away from the wall and walk your hands toward the wall till they are a foot away from the wall or closer. Keep at it, till you are able to perform 20-30 walk ups. Before this is achieved, you should continue to perform shoulder presses with feet on the chair.

When the hand stand walk up is mastered, you may start practicing the negatives and go from there as is outlined in the body press chapter on page 32.

The last photo in this chapter demonstrated the handstand press with the back toward the wall. In some cases this is a safer option for a beginner.

Free standing hand stand press is beyond the scope of this book. For this reason it is necessary to have a wall. Most people have difficulty standing up once they have performed a set of hand stand presses, if their body is facing the wall. This is one of the reasons why it is important to master the handstand walk up. The hand stand walk up allows you to safely get into the handstand position and safely get out of it. If however you still feel the need for rear support, or want to try a new variation all you have to do is face the wall, place you hands on the floor and kick you feet over.

Since this is the third exercise in the sequence it requires no separate warm up. Go ahead, build strong shoulders, so that the world can rest effortlessly on them.

Incline Push Ups

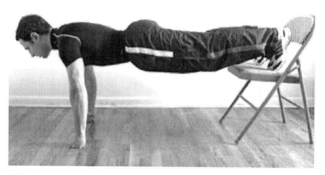

Pic. 1

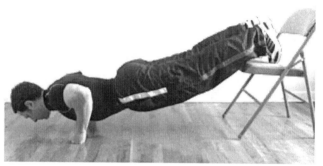

Pic. 2

- **Action:** Assume a push up position. Place your feet on the chair or other object of the relative height. (Pic. 1) Lower your chest to the floor. (Pic. 2) Press back up.
- **Key points:** Keep the abdominals and gluts squeezed, to protect the back. Keep the body in straight line.
- **Purpose:** To begin the progression sequence leading up to hand stand press.

Inclined Triangle Push Ups

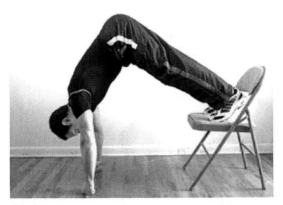

Pic. 1

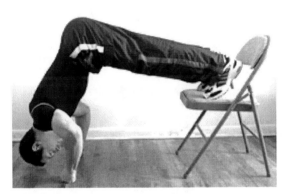

Pic. 2

- **Action:** Assume the previous position. Walk you hands about a foot toward the chair. (Pic. 1) Perform the push ups. (Pic. 2)
- **Key points:** Keep the abdominals tight to protect the back.
- **Purpose:** To transfer the work from the chest to the shoulders.

Shoulder Press Push Ups

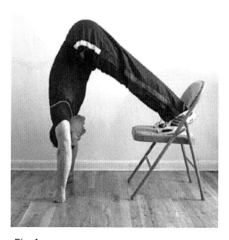

Pic. 1

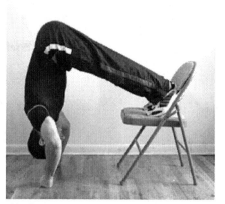

Pic. 2

- **Action:** Assume the previous position. Walk your hands toward the chair till the trunk is relatively vertical. (Pic. 1) Perform the pressing movement. (Pic. 2)
- **Key points:** Keep the abdominals tight to protect the back.
- **Purpose:** To practice similar movement to a handstand press, using less resistance.

Single Leg Shoulder Press

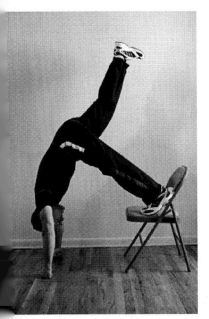

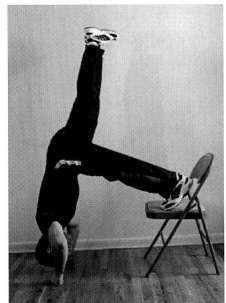

1

Pic. 2

- **Action:** Assume the previous position. Lift one leg up. (Pic.1) Perform the pressing movement. (Pic.2)
- **Key points:** Keep the abdominals tight to protect the back.
- **Purpose:**To provide additional resistance to the previous exercise.

Hand Stand Walk Up

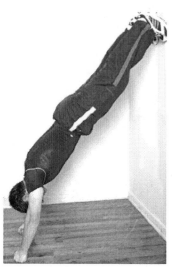

Pic. 1

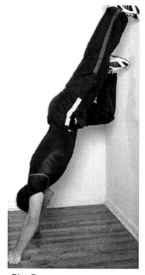

Pic. 2

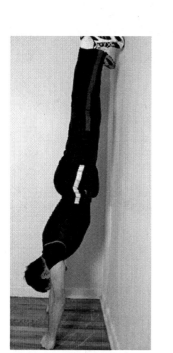

Pic. 3

- **Action:** Place your hand on the floo— few feet away from the wall. Pla your feet on the wall. (Pic. 1) W your hands toward the wall, as y feet climb up the wall. (Pics 2-3) turn to the staring position.
- **Key points:** Keep the abdomin tight. Take small steps.
- **Purpose:** To strengthen the core bilizers. To appreciate the feel for dynamic upside-down posture.

Hand Stand Press

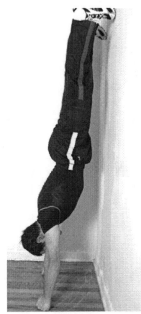

Pic. 1

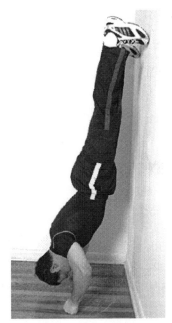

Pic. 2

- **Action:** Place your hand on the floor a few feet away from the wall. Place your feet on the wall. Walk your hands toward the wall, as your feet climb up the wall, till the body is vertical. (Pic.1) Lower your head toward the floor. (Pic. 2)Press back up.
- **Key points:** Keep the abdominals tight. Perform the movement slowly.
- **Purpose:** To strengthen the muscles, used for over head pressing.

Hand Stand Press (Back to the Wall)

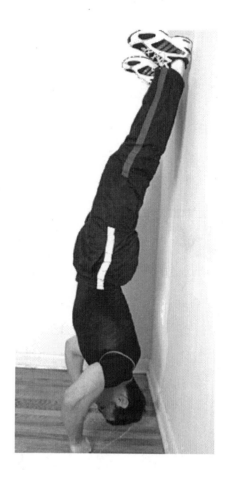

- **Action:** Face the wall. Place your hands on the floor approximately a foot away from the wall. Kick the feet up and over. Once in a handstand proceed to pressing motion.
- **Key points:** Keep the abdominals tight.
- **Purpose:** To provide another variation of the handstand press.

ROCKET

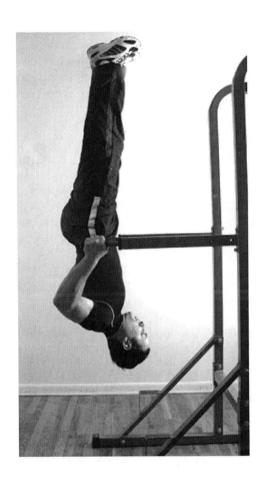

Rocket is a unique exercise. It strengthens the shoulders and upper back as well as elbow flexors. It balances out the muscles developed by the dips.

As you know by now the whole ElasticSteel Method (If you haven't read my other books The ElasticSteel Method of Athletic conditioning & The Gravity Advantage Book, go to www.ElasticSteel.com to get them), including the GAM is deeply rooted with the principles of balance.

Rocket complements the dips. Dips is a great exercise, but when left unbalanced it can lead to bad posture, and functional musculoskeletal disturbance will follow.

At the same time this exercise strengthens the shoulders in a totally different way. Not only does it sculpt and strengthen shoulders, it adds strength in previously unfamiliar territory of movement. For sports which are unpredictable and everything is possible, this is an absolute must. Those sports include, wrestling, football, martial arts, gymnastics. Same can be applied to occupations with potential surprises such as bouncers, fire fighters, soldiers.

Balance is an essential factor to have, prior to working on the strength element of this technique. First and foremost you must be able to hold yourself in the inverted vertical position. Three factors need be present for this to happen. You need a strong grip. You need an awareness of space and you need circulation. Yes, circulation. In other words, if you are not used to spending time upside down, than you may get light headed. This is the last thing you need, when you are upside down.

Grip is also very essential. If you can't hang in the upright position (Pull up position), most likely you will not be able to hang in the inverted position. I don't have to tell you what can happen when you are upside down, and you loose your grip. For this reason please; make sure that the bars are stable. Make sure that they can support your body weight easily. Last, but not least, make sure that you have a strong grip and can get out of the position in an instant if you happened to loose the grip.

Once you have established the grip, you may begin the inverted hang. Be careful; always be ready to drop your legs in the same direction of where they came from. If your legs begin to drop in the opposite direction, make sure to reverse that.

If at any point you feel like you are loosing balance, quickly bend your knees and return your feet to the floor.

It is recommended that you master the inverted hang, prior to moving on. You should be able to hang for at least 30-60 seconds, struggle free and completely vertical.

At this point you may begin to work on the negatives. Starting with the arms bent and slowly extending your arms and lowering the body. At the same time, as you are working on the negative, try the decline row. This exercise is easier than the rocket due to stability. Decline row is also a close relative of the more familiar, body row. Since a decline row is required to set up for the eccentric rocket movement, you should practice the row after the rocket negatives. In other words if you practice the decline row first, you won't have enough strength to lift yourself up in preparation for the negative rockets.

Once you have achieved one negative begin practicing the up and down movement of this exercise. Refer to page 32.
Follow the same protocol listed for the body press.

Go build you shoulders!

Inverted Hang

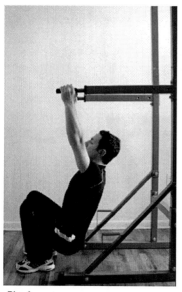

Pic. 1

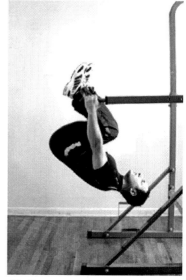

Pic. 2

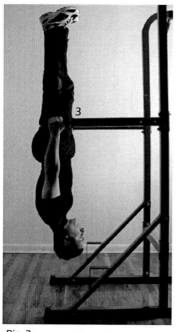

Pic. 3

- **Action:** Grip the bars with b hands, keeping the arms strai Bend the knees. (Pic. 1) Lean b and elevate your lower body. (Pi Extend the legs straight up. (Pic Return to the starting position in verse order.
- **Key points:** Make sure the bars handle the body weight, and gri secure.
- **Purpose:** To develop the awarer of the body, while in the upside-d position.

Decline Body Rows

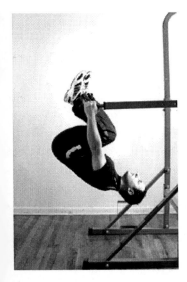

Pic. 1

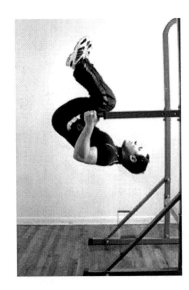

Pic. 2

- **Action:** Assume the decline body row position. (Pic.1) Pull yourself up. (Pic. 2) Return to the starting position.
- **Key points:** Try to maintain the trunk at an angle toward the ground, through the exercise.
- **Purpose:** To provide a transition, from the rowing action to the rocket pulling action.

Rocket (Negative Movement)

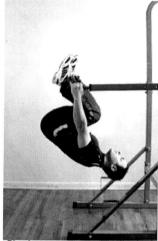

Pic. 1

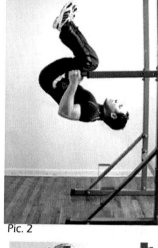

Pic. 2

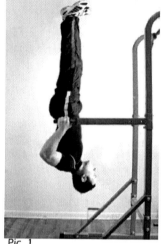

Pic. 1

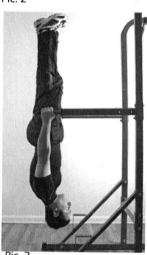

Pic. 2

- **Action:** Begin by assuming the decline body row position. (Pic. 1) Pull your body up as much as possible. (Pic. 2) Keeping the arms flexed assume the rocket position. (Pic. 3) Hold for as long as possible. Slowly extend the arms. (Pic. 4) Repeat all steps.
- **Key points:** As the arms extend in the rocket position, focus on keeping the body perfectly vertical.
- **Purpose:** To build up the strength to perform the rocket, by using negative movement.

Rocket

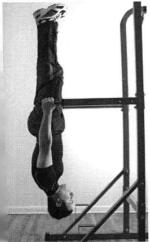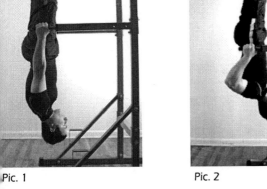

Pic. 1   Pic. 2

- **Action:** Assume a straight arm rocket position. (Pic. 2) Flex the arms, pulling your body upward. (Pic. 2) Return to the starting position.
- **Key points:** Focus on keeping the body perfectly vertical.
- **Purpose:** To strengthen the muscle groups used in performing the rocket.

RESOURCE

If you haven't yet read my other two books The ElasticSteel Method of Athletic Conditioning or The Gravity Advantage Book, and would like to get your hands on them. Go to www.ElasticSteel.com, don't forget to sign up to the forum, there's a wealth of information available there.

PULL UPS

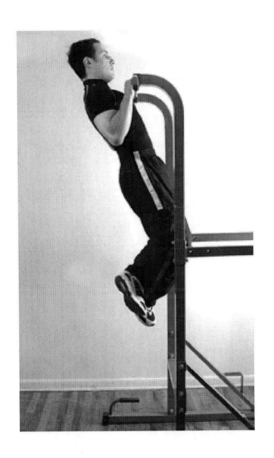

The pull up is known as the king of back development. It comes fifth in the sequence of the upper body exercises. If you are able to do the pull ups, pat yourself on the back, and go do them. If you can't, please follow the sequence of progression and you will be able to.

For those of us who don't know the difference between pull ups and chin ups, here it is. The grip for the pull ups is pronated or palms away from you. The grip for the chin ups is supinated or palms toward you. If you are using a straight bar than feel free to go from one exercise to another. If the dipping bar is high enough, the pull up can be performed on them as well. Both pieces of equipment would be used in this book to demonstrate the sequence of progression.

First, pull ups is performed with the assistance of a squat. The key to success here is force distribution. You can use the legs more than the arms, or the other way around. It's up to you. As you can guess, the arms should do most of the work. Leg work should be minimal and only as much absolutely necessary. Since cheating is possible the goal should be not so much on number of reps, but rather on the minimal use of the legs.

Single leg variations is more of a test, then progression. If you are able to pull mostly with your legs, then it doesn't make a difference if it's one leg on the floor or two. If indeed you have struggle with one leg off the floor, you know that more upper body strength is needed.

A chair suspended pull up is the next step. This exercise allows you a limited use of lower body support. Since it's difficult to cheat with this exercise, you should have an aim. Focus on working your way up to 3 sets of 15-20 repetitions.
Once you have reached that goal. Begin working on the negative or eccentric pull ups. You may use a chair or a jump to get yourself into the flexed arms position. Hold your arms flexed for as long as possible and slowly extend them. People who start working on eccentric pull ups without any prior preparation, such as suspended chair pull ups, are up for quite bit of struggle. On the other hand if you have spent time diligently practicing the suspended chair pull ups, you should be able to transfer the negatives into complete pull ups after some training.

Once you have achieved one pull up, refer to page 32 for increasing the number of repetitions.

Squat Assisted Pull Ups

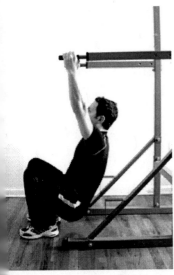 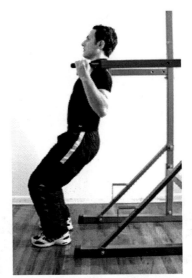

Pic. 1
Pic. 2

- **Action:** Grip the Dipping bars with both hands. Your feet should remain flat on the floor. (Pic. 1) Pull yourself up. (Pic. 2) Return to the starting position.
- **Key points:** Use the arms as much as possible. Legs should only provide the minor assistance.
- **Purpose:** To strengthen the muscles used for pull ups via the assistance of the legs.

Single Leg Squat Assisted Pull Ups

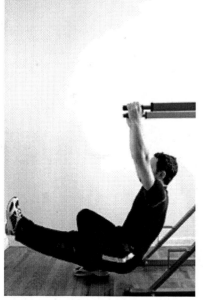 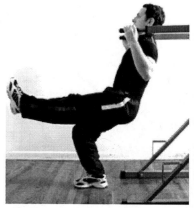

Pic. 1   Pic. 2

- **Action:** Assume the same position as the previous exercise. Extend one leg. (Pic. 1) Pull yourself up. (Pic. 2) Return to the starting position.
- **Key points:** Allow your legs to provide only a necessary assistance to the pulling action of the arms.
- **Purpose:** To strengthen the muscles used for pull ups.

Chair Suspended Pull Ups

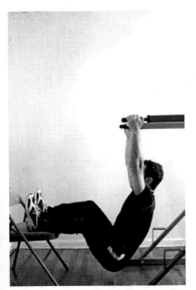

Pic. 1

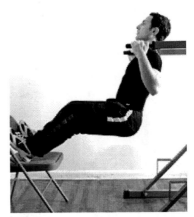

Pic. 2

- **Action:** Grip the dipping bars as if the pull up is about to be executed. Place the legs on the chair. (Pic. 1) Perform the pull up. (Pic. 2)
- **Key points:** Let the arms lead the exercise, while the legs assist.
- **Purpose:** To strengthen the muscles used in chin ups/ pull ups.

Jump Assisted Pull Up

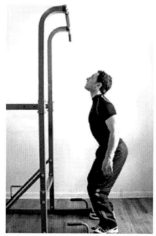

Pic. 1

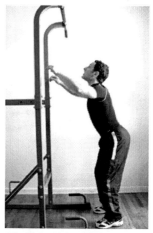

Pic. 2

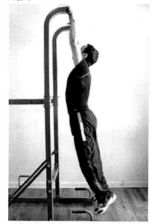

Pic. 3

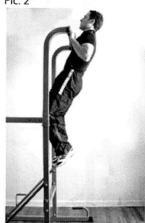

Pic. 4

- **Action:** Begin by standing in under and in front of the bar. Slowly aim and swing your arms back. (Pic. 1) Jump up and grip the bar, as the moment continues to displace you upward. (Pics 2-3) Use the acceleration of the legs to pull yourself up. (Pic. 4) Repeat the whole sequence.
- **Key points:** Catch the bar before the momentum is completely used up.
- **Purpose:** To use the moment of the jump, in order to execute a pull up.

DIPS

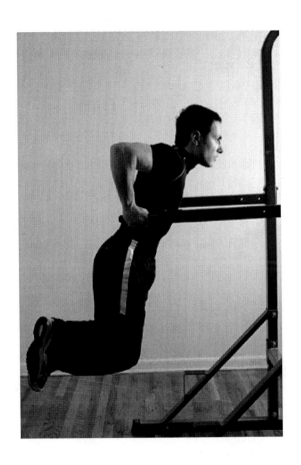

Dips is usually the least challenging exercise, thus it is placed last in the sequence. Depending on its variation it is the most commonly used body weight exercise to develop chest and/or triceps. When the body is properly prepared for this exercise, the results are usually quick to come by without any side effects. On the other hands many people push their body to perform dips, injuring themselves in the process. Dips are tough on the elbows, shoulders and the sternum. Many people complain of elbow pain, shoulder pain, and cracking sternum, as the result of performing dips.

Luckily above injuries can be avoided with preparation and proper techniques. In the matter of fact, even people who have avoided dips for years, can safely perform them, if they have had adequate preparation.

The dip progression is similar to the handstand progression to a large degree. Both exercise start with push ups and than slowly move away from them, while increasing the percentage of the body weight being lifted. While the handstand press moves the pressing movement overhead, the dips sequence moves the arms downward toward the hips, from the standard push ups.

Decline push ups is the first exercise in the sequence.
This action of this technique is slightly more downward than the regular push ups, thus recruiting the lower chest. Since the lower chest is larger and stronger than the upper, it is very likely that you will be able to do more repetitions of decline push ups, than regular or incline push ups. As you perform this exercise, try to focus on keeping your shoulder blades squeezed together throughout the repetitions. 3 sets of 20-30 repetitions, will be enough to move on.

Cobra dips is a variation of the decline push ups. It is designed to simulate the dips more than the previous exercise. Unlike the decline push ups, the body is arched, when the cobra dips are performed. On the concentric (upward) movement, the feet slide forward. This allows the trunk to remain more vertical, thus simulating the actual dipping motion. the feet slide on the floor backward, as you lower yourself down, between the chair.

Once in a while the surface of the floor or the friction of the shoes does not allow for sliding backward. In this case you will have to take small steps back with you feet, as your arms lower your body down. Any exercise involving the arching of the back, has a potential risk. To minimize that risk, remember to relax your hip flexors. (The muscles that are located in front of you hips. They lift you knee to perform a knee strike or the front kick.) Also remember to squeeze your buttocks and keep the abdominals tensed.

Once you feel comfortable with the cobra dips, you may move on to the chair assisted dips or the squat assisted dips. Once again, just like the chair assisted pull ups, use the legs as little as possible. Focus on lifting as much as possible with the arms, rather than focusing on the number of repetitions. You can cheat and perform many dips with the use of legs. On the other hand you can do only few reps, pressing with the arms to your full capacity.

Shrug downs are next. This exercise is designed to strengthen the muscles of the shoulder girdle. Strengthening the muscles that depress the scapula, will ensure the proper form when it's time to perform the dips. Shrug downs also strengthen the wrist. Having the wrist getting used to supporting the whole weight will prevent the premature termination of dips, due to weak wrist. In other words the wrist will not and should not be a limiting factor to how many dips you can do. As you work on this exercise continue to work on the chair assisted dips.

When you feel ready just like with other exercises, begin working on the negative dips. Follow the chart on page 32, for the instruction on increase the number of repetitions.

At his point you have discovered the six body weight exercises that you can use to super strengthen and develop you upper half.

Great luck to you!

Decline Push Ups

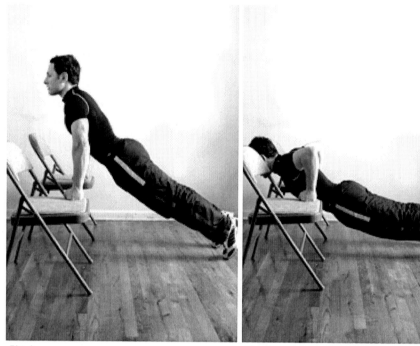

Pic. 1   Pic. 2

- **Action:** Assume a push up position with hands on the chairs. (Pic. 1)   Perform a push up. (Pic. 2)
- **Key points:** Keep the abdominals tight. Do now allow your lower back to over arch.
- **Purpose:** To prepare the body for the dipping motion.

Cobra Dips

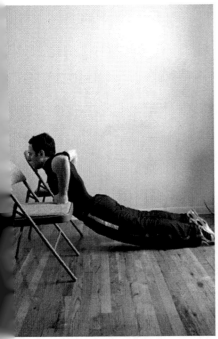

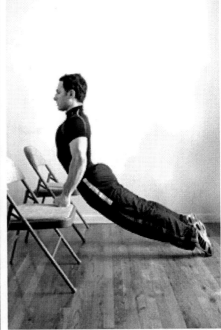

c. 1

Pic. 2

- **Action:** Assume a push up position with hands on the chairs. Arms bend. The body is curved backward. (Pic. 1) Keeping the body curved, push up. Your feet will drag forward slightly. (Pic. 2) Repeat.
- **Key points:** Keep the gluts tight. Allow the feet to move forward as you push up. Allow the feet to slide back as your lower yourself down.
- **Purpose:** To produce a downward pressing movement more than a regular declined push up can do.

Squat Assisted Dips

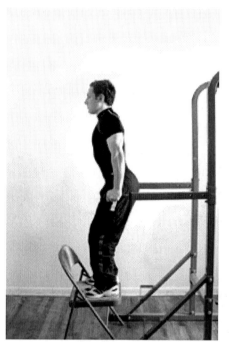 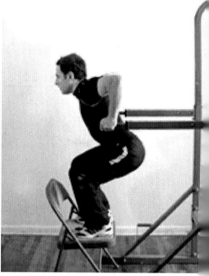

Pic. 1   Pic. 2

- **Action:** Stand up on the chair and assume a dipping position. (Pic. 1) Perform a dip. (Pic. 2)
- **Key points:** Concentrate on arms doing most of the work.
- **Purpose:** To prepare the body for the full force dipping motion.

Shrug Down

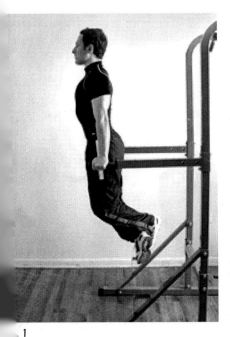 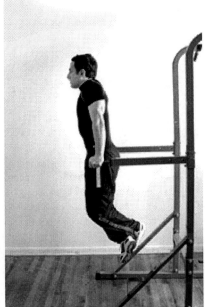

1   Pic. 2

- **Action:** Assume the straight arm dipping position. Shoulders are down and away form the ears. (Pic. 1) Keeping your arms straight, shrug and allow the shoulders to come up to the ears. (Pic. 2) Return to the starting position.
- **Key points:** Keep the arms soft; do not lock them out.
- **Purpose:** To strengthen the shoulder girdle muscles used in stabilization, while dips are performed.

Dips

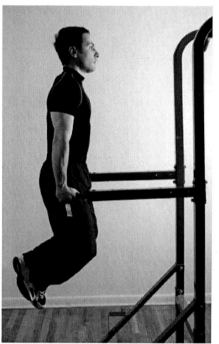

Pic. 1

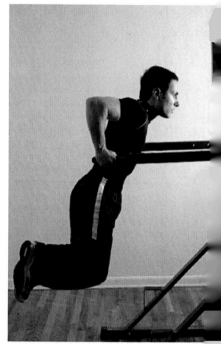

Pic. 2

- **Action:** Assume a dipping position. (Pic.) Flex the arms and lower yourself down. (Pic. 1) Return to the starting position.
- **Key points:** Keep the head up.
- **Purpose:** To strengthen the muscles used while dips are executed.

ONE-LEG SQUATS

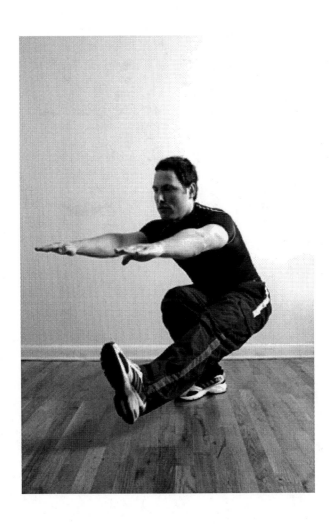

One leg squats have become a trade mark of the body weight exercising. For a trained athlete, who has never done one leg squat, mastery of this exercise is more about balance than strength. For most people however it's a combination of both factors. In sports where balancing yourself on one leg can make or break a champion squatting on one leg is rather common. Figure skaters rely on them for conditioning, so do gymnasts and certain dance stylists. One leg squat is also an important part of conditioning among skiers, and speed skaters. In addition to that many of the track athletes have begun to incorporate this technique into their training.

Single leg squat, depending on its variation hits the leg muscles harder than the regular squat. Most muscles lift double the load when the one leg squat is performed. Some muscle such as gluts get more than twice the resistance, due to greater work load caused by the shifted relation of center of gravity in relation to base of support. You will notice that your body will tend to shift side way to allow the standing leg to move inward to the center of mass.

Before you can squat on one leg, you must obviously be able to squat with both legs. Work your way up to 3 sets of 20-30 repetitions.

Once the basic squat is mastered, the chair is next. Chair is a static exercise. It helps to develop a single leg squat in two ways. Number one, by keeping the feet together, you better simulate a one leg squat. Second, it's the bend leg position that is often the most challenging. In other words, most people can squat down a little bit on one leg, but the further down they go, the more difficult it becomes. Leading from that it is important to develop strength, while the legs are bent. Chair positions helps with that. Aim at comfortably holding this position for at least one to two minutes.

While working on your minute mark, you may want to begin practicing the suspended leg squat. Although this exercise is performed with a one leg, it is less challenging than the single leg squat.

Once you can hold a chair for a minute or two, lift one foot an inch off the floor. This is the one leg chair. Work on being able to hold this position for 30 seconds on each leg.

After half a minute has been achieved, extend the non-supported leg. This will help if you want to do a one leg squat with the non squatting leg straight. Keeping the leg straight looks nicer, but is not necessary. In fact, bending the leg slightly should make the exercise easier.

Now here is an interesting point about the one leg squat. While most exercises are trained with negative first, this exercise is often started with positive movement first. Most people struggle to establish balance as they squat down on one leg, thus failing to complete the descent. However once you are in the bottom position, you have the balance already established, while standing one leg, it's only a matter of strength to be able to stand up. Keeping that in mind, we can assume that the previous exercises have already built up your strength, so you will be able to straighten your supporting leg and stand up.

If you still have trouble with this exercise, chair assisted one leg squats may be of help to you. Just make sure to ascend and descend very slowly using the strength of your muscles and not the momentum.

The last two exercises are added for variation. The first variation allows you to rest the hip flexor muscles, which hold the non squatting leg in front of you. Also by holding the leg behind, slightly different muscles are recruited. Since the body is forced to bend forward more, the lower back and the hamstrings are placed under greater functional stress.

If you have a pole or a stick available you can add more challenge to the one leg squat by manually pressing down on the lifted leg. It doesn't look too difficult, but when sufficient pressure is applied, the number or repetitions is drastically reduced.

Have fun squatting!

Squat

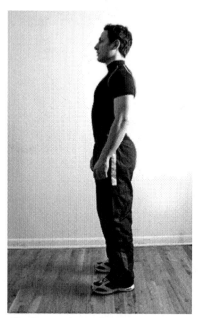

Pic. 1

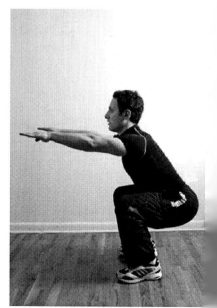

Pic. 2

- **Action:** Stand with your feet shoulder width apart. (Pic. 1) Extend your arms forward and squat down. Keep your head up and back straight. (Pic. 2) Return to the starting position.
- **Key points:** Keep the abdominals squeezed. Do not allow your toes to go past the knees.
- **Purpose:** To prepare the leg muscles for the more advanced leg exercises.

Chair

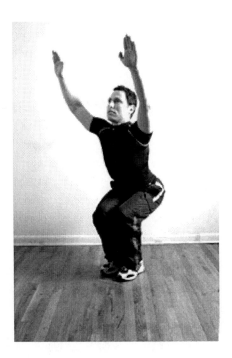

- **Action:** Place your feet together or few inches apart. Squat down and raise your arms over your head. Hold this position for as long as comfortable.
- **Key points**: Keeping the back straight lean forward from the waist slightly. Do not allow your knees to go pass our toes.
- **Purpose:** To strengthen the muscle required to perform the single leg squat.

Suspended Leg Squat

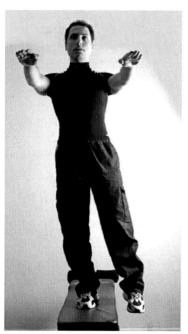

Pic. 1

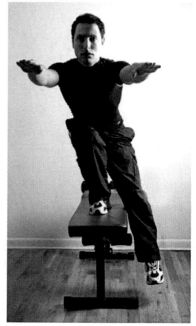

Pic. 2

- **Action:** Stand on a bench or a chair. Lift one leg slightly to the side. (Pic. 1) Squat down till the knee is at a 90 degree angle. (Pic. 2) Return to the starting position.
- **Key points:** Do not let the knee go past the toes.
- **Purpose:** To develop the strength and balance required to perform a single leg squat.

One leg chair

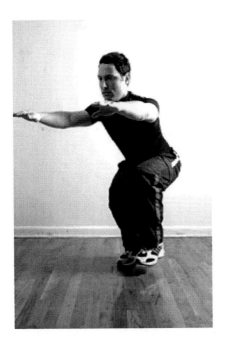

- **Action:** Assume the squat/chair position. Lift one leg slightly of the ground. Hold for as long as possible. Switch legs.
- **Key points:** Hold the position for the same amount of time on both side.
- **Purpose:** To develop unilateral static strength and balance.

One leg chair (Straight leg)

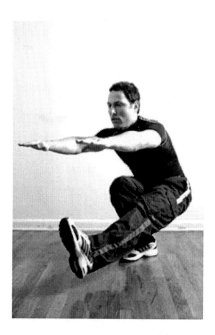

- **Action:** Assume the previous position. Extend the lifted leg. Hold for as long as possible. Switch legs.
- **Key points:** Hold the position for the same amount of time on both side.
- **Purpose:** To develop unilateral static strength and balance in preparation for the single leg squat.

Chair Assisted Single Leg Squat

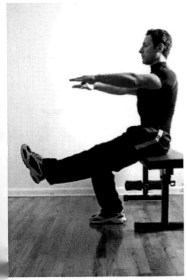

Pic. 1

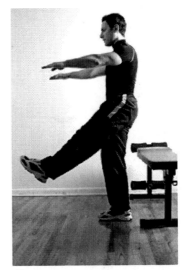

Pic. 2

- **Action:** Have a seat on the bench or a chair. Raise your arms forward. Lift one leg up. (Pic. 1) Stand up, while keeping the arms and legs in the same position. (Pic. 2) Return to the starting position.
- **Key points:** Keep the abdominals tight. Do not allow momentum to carry the movement.
- **Purpose:** To strengthen each leg unilaterally.

Single Leg Squat

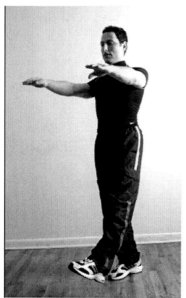

Pic. 1

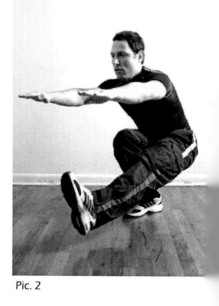

Pic. 2

- **Action:** In standing position raise your arms up. Lift the leg forward slightly. (Pic. 2) Squat down. (Pic. 2) Return to the starting position.
- **Key points:** Move the hips slightly to the side over the supporting (standing) leg.
- **Purpose:** To strengthen the muscles of the leg.

Single leg squat
Alternating leg forward and back.

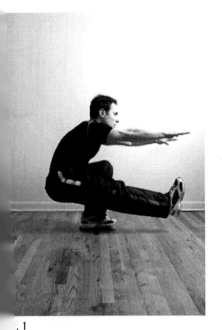 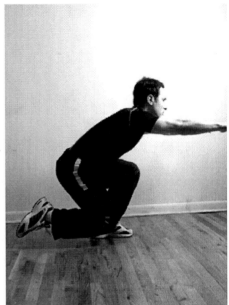

. 1   Pic. 2

- **Action:** Perform a single leg squat for one repetition. (Pic. 1) For the second repetition, fold the leg back and squat down. (Pic. 2) Continue to alternate between the two variations.
- **Key points:** Keep the supporting foot flat on the floor.
- **Purpose:** To give a variation to the single leg squat.

Manual Resistance Single Leg Squat.

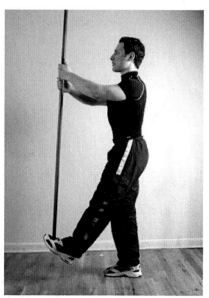

Pic. 1

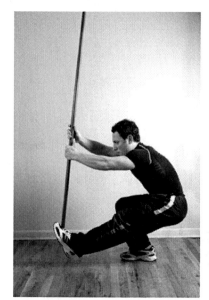

Pic. 2

- **Action:** Assume a starting position for a single leg squat. Place a stick between the instep and the toes. Apply downward pressure with your arms. (Pic. 1) Perform a single leg squat. (Pic. 2)
- **Key points:** Adjust the manual pressure as needed.
- **Purpose:** To increase the difficulty level of a single leg squat.

AIR LUNGES

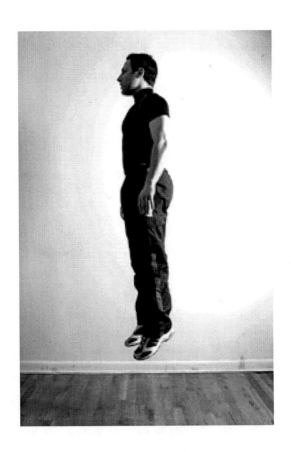

The air lunges give you everything you want from a complex multi joint leg exercise. Every major muscle in the leg is stressed. The exercise is very functional. Many factors necessary to athletic performance are developed. Some of those include, explosive strength, speed, balance, endurance, and power.

Air lunges is one of the most inclusive leg exercises. It develops every major muscle in the leg. It allows each leg to develop individual strength unilaterally. An athlete who competes on his feet, will benefit from this exercise.

The most common mistake that people make is rushing into this exercise. For an onlooker, the air lunges are easy technique to perform, and no preparation is needed. This is a wrong assumption. A number of factors must be considered prior to beginning this exercise.

Can you perform a perfect lunge? Does your front knee stay approximately over your foot? Can you keep your rear knee from slamming into the floor? Can you keep your body upright?
If you tested yourself and answer yes to all the questions, then you are partial ready for air lunges.

The second part has to do with strength. Your muscles and other tissue must be strong enough to take the impact of landing. In case this strength is not present, injuries can result, even if you have a proper lunging technique.

Due to above rationale the following is recommended. Begin by working on the front and back lunges. If you do the alternating sides (left leg, right leg, left leg, right leg) than you should be able to build up to at least 50 comfortable repetitions. If you do one side a time, than you should aim at 25 repetitions per leg. This applies to both front and rear leg lunges.

Once you have mastered the front and back lunge. Proceed to the air lunges. First few times you attempt this exercise, do not jump too high. Start with an inch or two height jump and slowly increase it.

Keep with this technique and watch your legs develop into powerful, functional machine.

Front Lunge

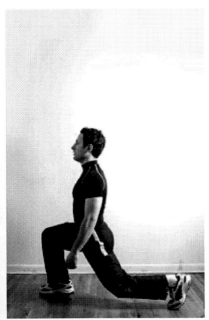

Pic. 1

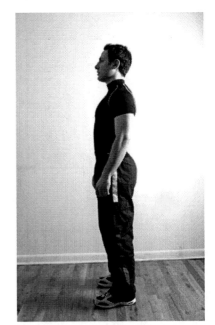

Pic. 2

- **Action:** Stand upright, feet shoulder width apart. Arms hanging loose by your sides. (Pic. 1) Step forward with one leg, until the other knee is almost touching the ground.(Pic. 2) Return to the starting position. Repeat on the other side.
- **Key points:** Do not allow the front knee to pass the toes.
- **Purpose:** To prepare for the air lunge.

Back Lunge

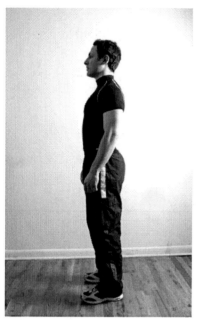

Pic. 1

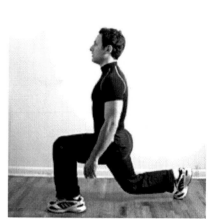

Pic. 2

- **Action:** Stand upright, feet shoulder width apart. Arms hanging loose by your sides. (Pic. 1) Step back with one leg, until the knee of the back leg is almost touching the ground. (Pic. 2) Return to the starting position. Repeat on the other side.
- **Key points:** Step back far enough so that the rear knee is below or behind the hips, not under the hips.
- **Purpose:**To prepare for the air lunge.

Air Lunges

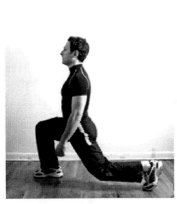

Pic. 1

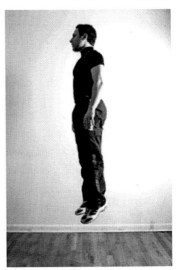

Pic. 2

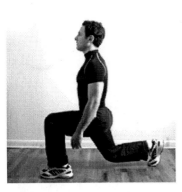

Pic. 3

- **Action:** Lunge forward. (Pic. 1) Jump straight up and bring your feet together. (Pic. 2) As you are landing, switch the legs. Land in the lunge position with the opposite leg in front. (Pic. 3) Repeat.
- **Key points:** Be careful not to bump the knee into the floor.
- **Purpose:** To develop strength, balance and explosiveness in the legs.

DRAGON CURL

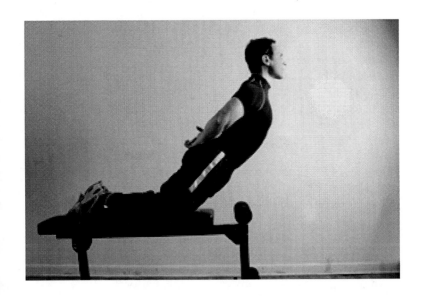

Dragon curl is the king of posterior chain exercises. When properly done, it develops unmatchable strength in the muscle running along the back of the legs and back of the trunk. In modern times the usual emphasis has been on the mirror muscles. In other words, if you can't see them in the mirror, you don't train them. Abdominals are worked hard, while the extensors of the spine are neglected. Many common exercises drill quadriceps and neglect hamstrings.

Worst yet, it is very common not only to forgo building posterior chain strength, but to focus on constantly lengthen it. Think about it; what are the most common stretches for? Hamstrings, gluts, lower back calves. This leads to imbalance.

Based on the reason stated above, you will understand why Dragon Curl has a very long sequence of progression. Most people are simply not ready to perform this exercise. This even refers to people who have been working on their leg muscles.

Prior to going any further let's take a quick look at the anatomy of the posterior chain. Two of the posterior chain muscle groups work over two joints each. Hamstrings flex the knee and extend the hip. In other words, they pull the heel toward the gluts, thus bending the knee. Hamstrings also extend the hip angle along with gluts such as in dead lift or front leg during lunge. Calf muscles perform two actions as well. They point the toes, such as in toe raisers and they bend the knee, just like hamstrings do.

That being said you can guess that the dragon curl requires such a long progression sequence. Most people train the prime movers of this exercise, but not over the right joints. The hamstrings are usually trained to extend the hip. This can be seen exercises such squat, lunge, dead lift, stiff leg dead lift, hyperextensions, leg press. The calf is usually trained to point the toes: calf raisers, toe press jumps, donkey presses. Not much training is done when it comes flexing the knee.

We begin by strengthening your lower back, and other back muscles running along your spine. Since back muscles are the stabilizers of this exercise, you can't possibly do without them. Start performing 2 sets of 20 Supermans. Work up to 3 sets of 30.

Once the above goal is achieved move on to hyper extensions. This exercise places a strong emphasis on your back, but recruits other posterior chain muscles as well.

Follow the repetitions and guidelines of the previous exercise. Starting with hyper extensions and forward, you must decide how you will secure your lower legs.

Two most common options are partner or ropes. If you decide to train with a partner make sure that it is someone who is available when you need him. At the same time, this person must be strong and preferably same weight as you or heavier. It is not easy to hold someone feet down, especially for a high number of repetitions.

For this reason I usually recommend some kind of device to hold the legs down. In the pictures a luggage strap is used. It is not expensive and does a fine job. You do have to test, how strong yours is first. If you looking for more comfort, weight lifting belt may be another option. It is wider and softer than the strap. Make sure you get a device which is easy to open and close, especially if you are going to be opening and closing it yourself. The good part is, if you ask someone open and close the belt or strap, that person doesn't have to be as strong as someone who will hold your legs in place.

Once you have mastered the hyper extension, cobra bends are next. This exercise continues to challenge the lower back, gluts and hamstrings. The point of this exercise is to activate the flexors of the knees. (Hamstrings, calves.) These muscles perform stabilizing, static contractions. They stabilized your thighs in the upright positions. The maximum stabilization force is required when the trunk is parallel to the floor. You may not be able to come down this low at first.

Start with leaning only slightly forward. Work your way down, till you can easily achieve a 90 degree angle at your hips. Ideally, your knee should stay at a 90 degree angle through this exercise. Work your way to 3 sets of 20 repetitions. Since this is type of movement is new to your body, start slowly. Depending on your overall conditioning, 2 sets of 5 may be a good starting point.

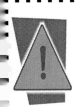

RESOURCE

Go to ElasticSteel.com and sign up to the forum where you can get all your GAM questions answered by your fellow GAM practitioners.

The next exercise is called the Let Down. It is an eccentric exercise. Here the lower back and gluts act as stabilizers, while the hamstrings act as prime movers. In reality, hamstrings work as decelerators. It is critical not to rush this exercise. Make sure that you have truly mastered the cobra bends prior to attempting this exercise. As you are learning the let down, be ready to place your hands on the floor and stop yourself from falling if necessary. Use a chair, bench or partner assistance to come back up.

At first you may not be able to control the movement, it's ok, stay with it. After some practice you will notice that you have more control when your knees are bent. As your legs become straighter, you begin to loose control. This is natural, don't fight it. With time it will improve. Keep in mind that while you practice this technique, you are indeed becoming stronger, your hamstrings and the whole posterior is getting more and more developed. Start with 2 sets of 5. Since this is an eccentric exercise the speed and control not quantity determines its mastery. One slow, controlled let down can be more meaning full, than 20 consecutive uncontrollable falls. While working on this exercise, continue to practice the cobra bend.

So far the routine should look like this.

<u>Warm up</u>

- 2 Sets of 10 squats
- 2 sets of 10 dead lifts (Stiff leg prepared.)
- 1 set of 10 hyper extensions.
- 1 set of 10 cobra bends.

<u>Work out</u>

- 2 set of 5 let downs. Increase to 3 sets of 10
- 3 sets of 20 cobra bends.

Again this is the sample work out for someone who has mastered the cobra bends and is now working on let downs and cobra bends. If you haven't mastered the cobra bends, do not begin practicing the let downs.

The next exercise in the Dragon Curl progression combines the Cobra Bends and Let Downs. It's called the Dragon-Cobra Bow. Obviously both previous exercises must be mastered before attempting the combination. The combination requires you to be able to hold yourself in half let down position, while performing the eccentric cobra bend. Following that you must hold the ninety degree angle at your hips, while flexing your knees from a 135 to a 90 degree angle. This is the first time that knees flex against resistance. Mastering the previous two exercises will ensure the success here. Finally, extend your trunk to a vertical position, as soon as the knees are at a 90 degree angle.

Once again this exercise is your first encounter, with true concentric movement in this preparatory sequence (Against the pull of gravity.). As you might have noticed already it is easier to begin flexing the knee when it is already bent, thus the reason for this exercise.

Start with 2 sets of 5. If you can only perform one or two, keep at it, till the number of repetitions increase. When you can perform 2-3 sets of 15-25 repetitions you are ready to move on.

Suspended Cobra Bends is the next challenge. This exercise requires both static and dynamic contractions from the hamstrings. Statically the hamstrings hold the upper leg flexed at 45 degree, assisted by the calves. At the same time, hamstrings together with gluts extend the hips. Back muscles are important stabilizers here as well. As with above exercise when you can do 2-3 sets of 15-25 repetitions, you are ready to move on.

Cancel Out, is the next exercise. Its name explains what happens to the hamstring during movement. As the knees extend, the hamstrings lengthen. At the same time the hip extends and the hamstrings shortens. In other words, the simultaneous action of the two joints, cancels each other out. One allowing the hamstring to become longer, the other doing the opposite and allowing the hamstring to become shorter. This exercise allows the hamstring muscle to experience the effect of the full torque at the complete knee extension.

The main point of this exercise is the eccentric movement (downward, toward gravity). Focus on slow controlled repetitions. Quality of each repetition is more important than the quality. The concentric movement (Returning back up to the starting position.) is usually assisted. A partner can help you up, or you can use a chair or a bench to come back to the starting position. Again, start with 2-3 sets of 5 and work up to 2-3 sets of 15-25.

Please keep in mind that there is no contradiction. Yes, quality beats quantity. Yes, one repetition performed slowly over the length of one minute is better than 100 reps, when you are just falling with out control.

To put all this together, it is important to understand that by practicing one repetition, per work out will not increase the quality. A few sets with many repetitions will increase quality. Thus I am telling you that you may need a high number of repetitions to develop quality at the end. Keep in mind that you are trying to get control of every single of those repetitions on your way down. Falling down 50 times, without any attempt for control will not do you much good.

The next exercise allows you to perform a full negative of the Dragon Curl, while not having to use full force for upward return to the starting position. This exercise is called Dragon Cobra. It is named that because an element of the Dragon Curl is present and so is the element of the Cobra Bends. The first portion of this exercise is the eccentric contraction of the hamstrings and calves as the knee joint extends. The middle part of the exercise is the flexion of the knee to a 90 degree angle. This is the first time, that the knee flexes from a straight line to right angle. In order to make this easier at first, the hips bend simultaneously. The double flexion of the hip and the knee, makes this exercise slightly less challenging than a the Dragon Curl. The last part of the movement is similar to Cobra Bends. As with previous technique 2-3 sets of 5 should be a good start. Build up to 15-25 repetitions.

Now it's the time for your hard work and effort to pay off. One of the most difficult body weight exercises is next, the majestic Dragon Curl. This move takes your posterior chain strength to the next level. You should be able to master the eccentric Dragon Curl very well. If not, please go back. Try every exercise in the sequence; find where you need to be and start from there.

If you can easily come down, but can't come back up yet, there are two ways of handling this. First is the assistance of a prop. I used the chairs for demonstration in this book. The second way is partial movement. Here is how it's done.

Begin the exercise by going by lowering your trunk only a few degrees. Stop yourself and come back up. You may notice that at first you can lower your self only10 degrees, any further will prevent you from coming back up. Spend some time with this angle. With time you should be able to lower yourself closer to the bench and have enough strength and control to come back up.   This is when you know that you have achieved something truly phenomenon.

The last exercise in this chapter is added for the ultimate challenge. This exercise is called the   posterior chain escalator.

It works every posterior muscle as a mover and as a stabilizer. Once you master this exercise, you will be in a tight circle of fitness elite.

Superman

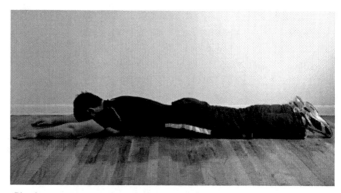

Pic. 1

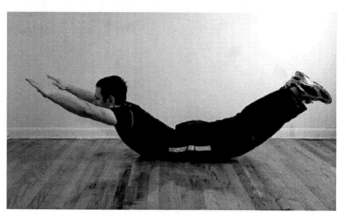

Pic. 2

- **Action:** Lie face down. Extend your arms and legs. (Pic. 1) Lift your arms and legs up. (Pic. 2) Hold for 3 seconds and return to starting position.
- **Key points:** Keep the left and right limb at equal height.
- **Purpose:** To strengthen the lower back, in preparation for the dragon curl.

Hyper Extension

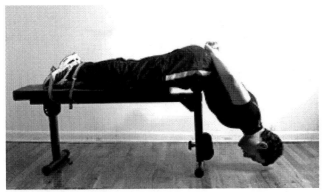

Pic. 1

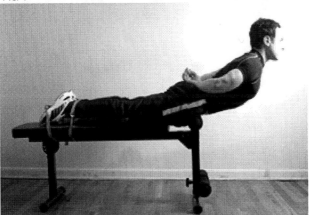

Pic. 2

- **Action:** Lie face down on the bench. Secure your lower leg to the bench. Bend forward at the hip level. (Pic. 1) Lift your torso as high as possible. (Pic. 2) Return to the starting position.
- **Key points:** Keep the back straight and shoulder blades squeezed together.
- **Purpose:** To strengthen the posterior chain in preparation for the dragon curl.

Cobra Bends

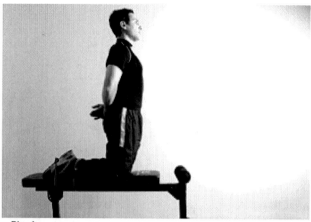

Pic. 1

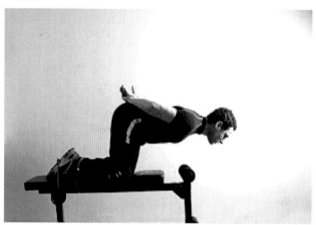

Pic. 2

- **Action:** Stand on your knees. Secure your feet to the bench or the floor. (Pic. 1) Keeping your thighs vertical, lean forward from the waste. (Pic. 2) Return to the starting position.
- **Key points:** Keep the abdominals squeezed. Keep the back straight.
- **Purpose:** To strengthen the posterior chain in preparation for the dragon curl.

Let Down

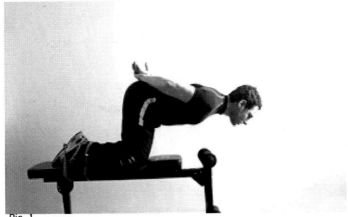

Pic. 1

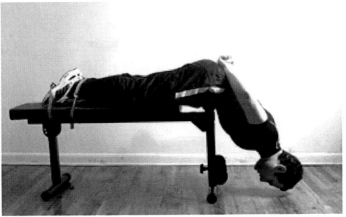

Pic. 2

- **Action:** Secure your feet. Stand on your knees and lean forward. (Pic. 1) Keeping your hips flexed, slowly extend your knees. (Pic. 2) Use your hands to guide you back into the starting position. Repeat.
- **Key points:** Keep the abdominal and gluts squeezed. Keep the back straight.
- **Purpose:** To strengthen the posterior chain in preparation for the dragon curl.

Dragon-Cobra Bow

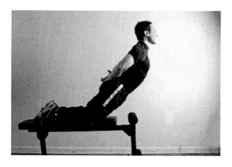

Pic. 1

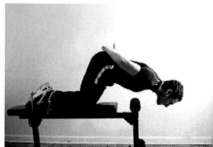

Pic. 2

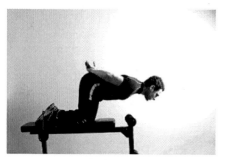

Pic. 3

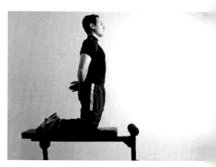

Pic. 4

- **Action:** Assume the kneeling position. Keeping the back straight tend your knees till the body is at a 45 degree angle. (Pic. 1) Keeping the thighs stable, lean forward from the hips. Once the hips rea 90 degree angle, stop. (Pic. 2) Keeping the hips at a 90 degree gle, contract the hamstrings and flex the knee, till the thighs are ve cal. (Pic. 3) Extend the hips and come up. (Pic. 4)
- Extend the hips and return to the upright kneeling position. Repea
- **Key points:** Keep the back straight. Protect the back, by holdin contraction in the gluts and abdominals.
- **Purpose:** To strengthen the posterior chain in preparation for dragon curl.

Suspended Cobra Bends

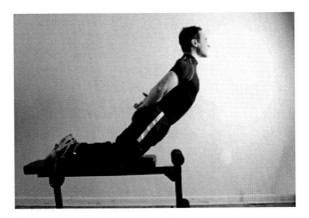

Pic. 1

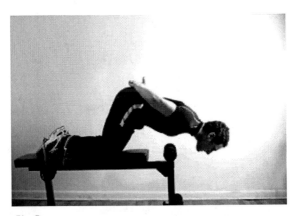

Pic. 2

- **Action:** Assume a kneeling position. Keeping the backs straight lean forward, till the body is at a 45 degree angle. (Pic. 1) Keeping the things stable at the 45 degree angle, lean forward till the hips are flexed at a 90 degree angle. (Pic. 2) Return to the starting position.
- **Key points:** Keep the back straight. Keep the gluts and abdominals tensed.
- **Purpose:** To strengthen the posterior chain in preparation for the dragon curl.

Cancel Out

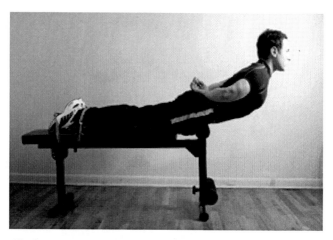

Pic. 1

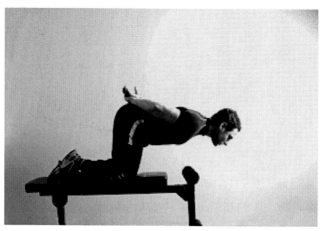

Pic. 2

- **Action: Secure your feet.** Lie face down. (Pic. 1) Flex the knees and hips at the same time. Come up to a 90 degree flexion of the hips and knees. (Pic. 2) Return to the starting position.
- **Key points:** Back straight. Gluts and abdominals are tensed.
- **Purpose:** To strengthen the posterior chain in preparation for the dragon curl.

Dragon Cobra

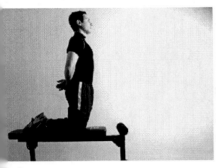

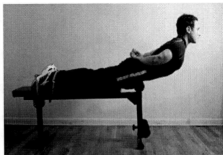

:. 1

Pic. 2

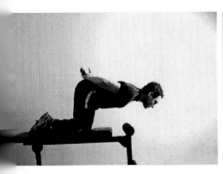

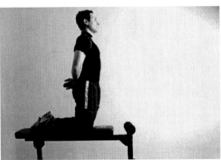

3

Pic. 4

Action: Assume the kneeling position. (Pic. 1) Slowly lower youself toward the bench. (Pic. 2) Flex your knees and hip at the same time, till both joints are at a 90 degree angle. (Plc. 3) Extend the hips and come up to a kneeling position. (Pic. 4) Repeat the sequence.
Key points: Keep the gluts and abdominal squeezed. Keep the back straight.
Purpose: To strengthen the posterior chain.

Assisted Dragon Curl

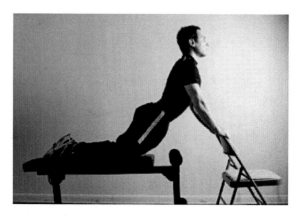

Pic. 1

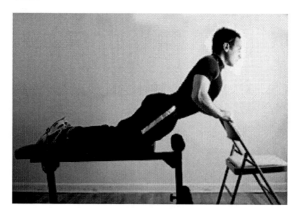

Pic. 2

- **Action:** Assume a kneeling position. Place your hands on a chair or another supporting object and extend your arms (Pic. 1) Relying minimally on the strength of your arms, lower yourself, by bending the arms.(Pic. 2) Return to the starting position.
- **Key points:** Use the arms only to guide the movement.
- **Purpose:** To develop the strength posterior chain in preparation for the dragon curl.

Dragon Curl

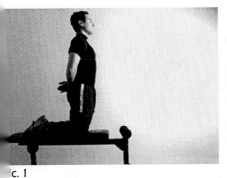

c. 1

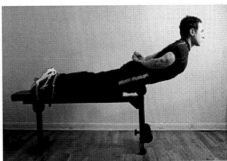

Pic. 2

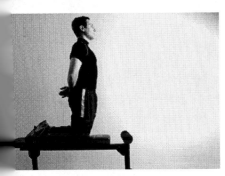

. 3

Action: Assume a kneeling position. (Plc. 1) Lower yourself toward the bench. (Pic. 2) Return to the starting position. (Pic. 3)

Key points: Keep your back straight. Squeeze the gluts and abdominals to protect the lower back.

Purpose: To develop the muscles in the posterior chain, including; the extensors of the spine, gluts, hamstrings and calves.

Posterior Chain Escalator

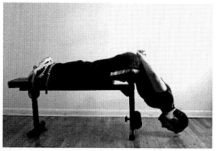

Pic. 1

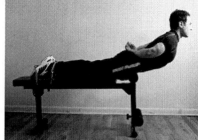

Pic. 2

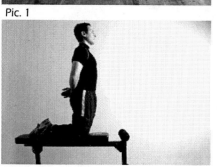

Pic. 3

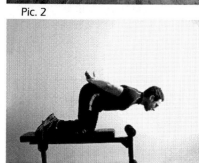

Pic. 4

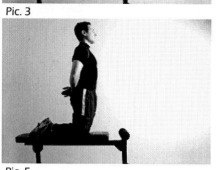

Pic. 5

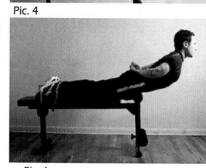

Pic. 6

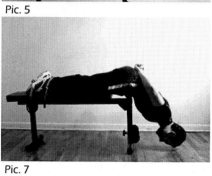

Pic. 7

L-EXTENSION
FLAG-EXTENSION

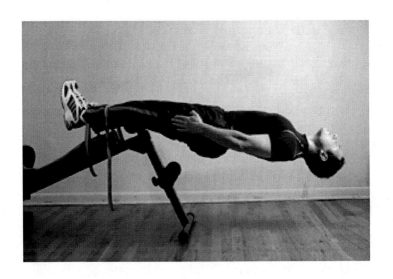

L-Extension is a body weight quadriceps strengthening exercise. Unlike squats, lunges and a variety of stances, the L-extension places the resistance load of the whole body on the front of the thigh. Many standard body weight quadriceps building exercise have to divide the lifting efforts between quadriceps, hamstrings and gluts. This exercise does not.

L-Extension also hits the lower quadriceps harder than do most other body weight exercise. Lower quadriceps are in close proximity to the knee as opposed to the hip.

This exercise gives your body a totally different feel for leg lower body training that most other training techniques. For martial arts practitioners, this is a great way to improve the power of the roundhouse and the front kick.

Like the Dragon curl, the L-extension is usually performed on the bench. A good, thick padding under the knees will ensure comfort during the execution of the technique. For this reason a sit up bench is usually chosen. If you do not have a partner, than you must have a bench where one end of the bench is steadily fixed. The L-Extensions are performed at the other end. The next requirement is the a belt or a strap, to stabilize the legs. In the photos a strap is used. It goes around the bench and your feet. Just make sure that it is strong enough to hold you. Having a partner, can lift the requirement of a fixed bench on one side. A partner can hold the free side of the bench down, by sitting on it. I do not recommend asking your partner to hold your legs down. This is a very difficult task. It will be difficult for you and the person who is holding down your legs.

Another variation of this exercise requires no equipment, but a strong partner that you trust. I did not demonstrate this variation, but will briefly describe it for informational sake. All the exercise can be performed on your partner shoulders. For this to be done you must place your legs over the trapezius and deltoid of your spotter. One of the ways to get into this position is to stand facing your partner, while his back is to you. Place your hands on the floor, get into the hand stand and kick your legs over your partner's shoulders. You are now upside down, you partner is upright and you backs are touching each other. You partner will have to adjust his height, so that his shoulders are at the level of the back of you knees, while you are in the hand stand. Once you bend your knees, and your feet are in front of your partner, he can grab your ankles and hold them down with his hands. Again, do this only with someone serious, experienced, strong and trustworthy.

With that said, let's begin. We begin by strengthening the abdominals and the hip flexors. Decline sit ups is the first exercise. It is more difficult than a regular sit up. Begin with 2 sets of 10 and build up to 3 sets of 15-25 repetitions. Another advantage of this exercise is that it helps your legs to adapt to the positions in which they are held.

Fulcrum seat is the next exercise. It involves holding the static contraction, while the legs are straight. This position may prove to be too challenging, if this is the case, feel free to assist yourself with manual support using chairs or other objects. Once you are able to maintain yourself in full suspension, begging timing yourself.   Make three attempts starting with 15-30 seconds each. Keep training till you are able to hold this position for a minute and a half (90 seconds) to two and a half minutes (150 seconds). Continue working on the decline sit up while practicing the fulcrum seat. Decline sit up should follow the fulcrum seat during your work out, when both are incorporated.

Once you are comfortable with the fulcrum seat you may begin working on the L-Extension. At first, guide yourself with outside support, such as chairs. Next, work on unassisted negatives and assisted positives. Again, quality is more important than the number or reps and sets.

Practice till you feel comfortable with these exercises, only then try the unassisted variation. Refer to page 32 for information on how to increase the number of repetitions.

If you haven't felt the challenge yet, that's about to change. Air Sit Up is next. This exercise is one of the most challenging body weight technique when it comes to the anterior chain. Air sit up forces every muscle located in front of your lower body and mid section to work as a team. There is no place for the weak link in this exercise. Always remember to protect your back, as you are performing air sit up. Squeeze your buttocks and your abdominals. Do not allow your lower back to over arch.

If you can't perform this exercise on the first try, don't despair. Assume a fulcrum seat and lean back only far enough that you can come back up. As you get stronger, you should be able to straighten you body more and more, till it is completely straight and parallel to the floor.

Like with other technique start the Air Sit up with 2 sets of five repetition. Build up to 3 sets of 15-25 repetitions. If you only perform 1 rep, take a loot at page 32.

Anterior chain escalator is the a combination of all the previous exercise in this chapter. It build a great endurance in your quadriceps, hip flexors, and abdominal. At the same time, it's one of the few exercise that trains all the muscles in your anterior chain to work together.

The last exercise in this sequence is the Flag Extensions. This exercise is as difficult as it looks. Due to effect of torque, Flag Extensions are the most difficult body weight quadriceps exercises. Rest assured, the hip flexors and abdominals are not off the hook of coarse, they work as hard as the next guy.

The best way to build up to Flag Extensions is to start with the L-Extensions and keep opening the hips as new level of strength is developed. To understand this better take a look at the starting position of the L-Extension. The upper body is upright. Now take a look at the starting position of the Flag extensions, the upper body is upside down.

The way to get from the L-Extensions to the Flag Extensions is to lower the trunk from the upright position to the upside down position few degrees at a time. If you are comfortable with the L-Extensions extend your hips, so that you body is on the 45 degrees incline. If this is too difficult, lean back only to the 10 or 15 degree incline and work your way down. Perform the leg extensions, while keeping your trunk at a comfortable angle. With time you should be able to keep your torso and thighs in one straight line, while only using the power of quadriceps to raise and lower your body. Don't make a mistake about it, your core will do allot of work, but it will all be static contractions.

Decline Sit Ups

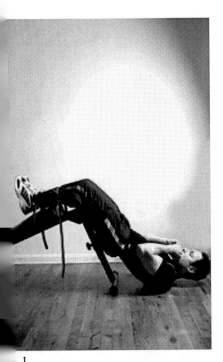

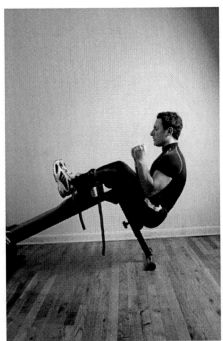

1   Pic. 2

Action: Place your lower legs on the bench. Secure the legs. (Pic. 1) Flex your hips and lift your upper body to an almost vertical position. (Pic. 2) Return to the starting position.
Key points: Keep the naval pulled in, to protect the lower back.
Purpose: To strengthen abdominals and hip flexors.

Fulcrum Seat

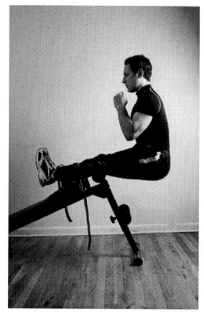

Pic. 1

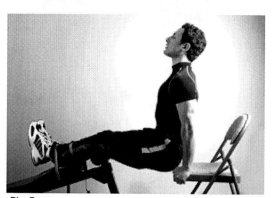

Pic. 2

- **Action:** Secure your lower legs on the bench. The padded edge of the bench should be right under and behind the knees. Keep the legs straight. Trunk upright.(Pic. 1) Chair can be used if support is needed. (Pic. 2)
- **Key points:** Keep the naval pulled in to protect the back.
- **Purpose:** To strengthen quadriceps, in fully shortened position, using isometric contraction.

Assisted L-Extension

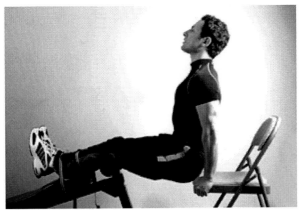

Pic. 1

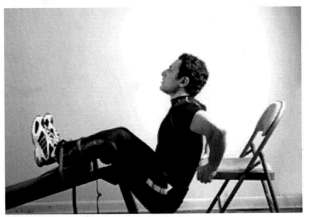

Pic. 2

- **Action:** Assume the previous position. Place your hands on the chair behind you. (Plc. 1) Relying mostly on the strength of your legs, lower your hips down. (Pic. 2)   Return to the starting position.
- **Key points:** Remember as the knees extend the hip travel up and away from the bench. If you are using a chair, make sure there is enough clearance for the hips to move away from the bench.
- **Purpose:** To strengthen the quadriceps.

L-Extension

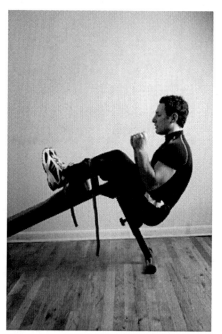

Pic. 1

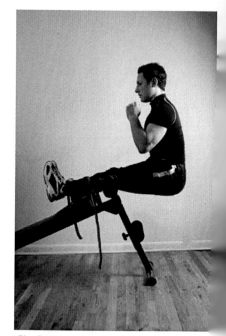

Pic. 2

- **Action:** Place your knees over the pads and secure the lower legs. (Pic. 1) Using the strength of the quadriceps extend the knees. (Pic. 2) Return to the starting position.
- **Key points:** Perform this movement slowly without bouncing.
- **Purpose:** To strengthen the quadriceps.

Air Sit Up

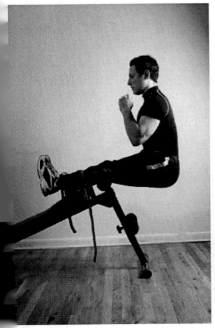

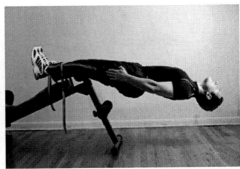

Pic. 1   Pic. 2

Action: Assume the previous position. (Pic. 1) Keeping the legs straight lean back. (Pic. 2) Return to the starting position.
Key points: The lower back must not be allowed to curve. Keep the gluts and abdominals squeezed throughout the movement.
Purpose: To strengthen the hip flexors, abdominals and other anterior chain muscles.

Anterior Chain Escalator

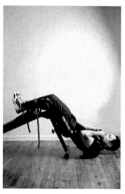

Pic. 1

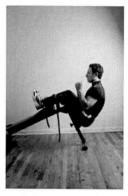

Pic. 2

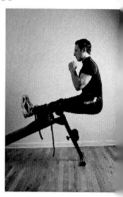

Pic. 3

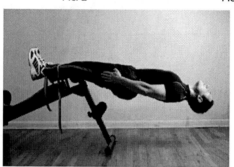

Pic. 4

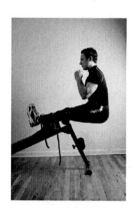

Pic. 5

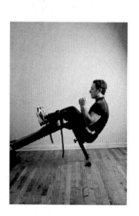

Pic. 6

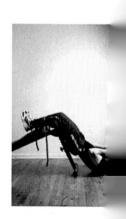

Pic. 7

Flag Extension

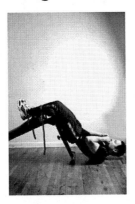

Pic. 1

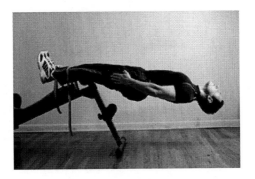

Pic. 2

- **Action:** Assume the decline sit up positon. (Pic. 1) Keeping the legs and upper body in one line, straighten your knees. (Pic. 2) Return to the starting position.
- **Key points:** . Keep the gluts and abdominals squeezed throughout the movement.
- **Purpose:** To strengthen the quadriceps and other anterior chain muscles.

SCISSORS PLANKS

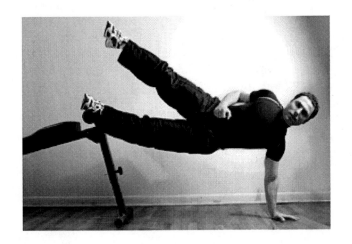

The last two exercises complete the program. So far all the technique were focused on forward and back movement. The closing scissors plank and the opening scissors plank work the "side to side" movers of the body. The closing scissors plank work the muscles located on the inner thigh. These muscles are responsible for bringing the leg toward the midline of the body. These are the same muscles being stretched, when one does a side split. Thus this exercise performed properly, helps in flexibility oriented conditioning. Strengthening the inner thigh will also prevent painful groin muscle pulls. The opening scissors plank is the opponent exercise to the close scissors plank. The former trains the muscles located on the outside of the hip. Developing this muscle group will help to develop quickness in lateral movements.

Besides strengthening the legs, both exercises strengthen the lateral stabilizers and flexors of the trunk. Lower back, abdominals, obliques, and quadratus lomborum greatly benefit from these exercises.

In relation to the whole program, the scissors planks are not as challenging as the other exercises. That being so, do remember that they will be performed last, when a lot of energy has been used up. Most people would be able to perform a few repetitions from the first try. If that is not the case try isometrically holding the starting or the ending position. If that proves too challenging, feel free to rest both legs on the bench, either isometrically or while performing the lateral flexion of the spine. Finally as a reminder, it's up to you to make this exercise as efficient as possible. To maximize the amount of work that legs perform compared to the midsection, try to keep your spine straight. The farther the spine flexes sideways, the more core muscles are stressed. Start with 2 sets of 5 and build up to 3 sets of 15-25. If this exercise does not provide enough challenge, feel free to increase the resistance. With your free hand place an item on your hip and hold it there throughout the exercise. Anything that can comfortably rest on our hip and has some weight would be suitable. You will see that it doesn't take a large increase in resistance to add a challenge and decrease the number of repetitions.

Closing Scissors Plank

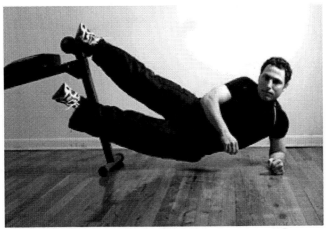

Pic. 1

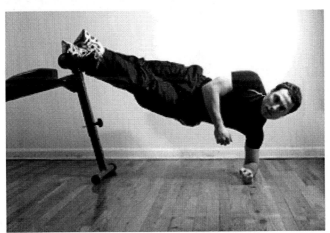

Pic. 2

- **Action:** Lie down on your side. Place the top leg on the bench or a chair. Support yourself with the bottom hand or the forearm. Lift your hips off the ground slightly. (Pic. 1) Raise your hips and your bottom foot at the same time. (Pic. 2) Return to the starting position.
- **Key points:** Keep the naval pulled in to protect the back.
- **Purpose:** To strengthen the inner thigh (adductors) and lateral flexors of the trunk.

Opening Scissors Plank

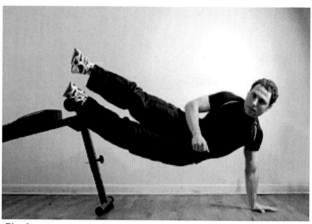

Pic. 1

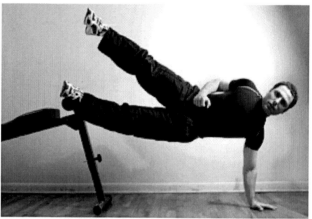

Pic. 2

- **Action:** Lie down on your side. Place the bottom leg on the bench or a chair. Support yourself with the bottom hand or the forearm. Lower your hips, as you stretch the hip muscles . (Pic. 1)   Raise your hips and the top foot at the same time. (Pic. 2) Return to the starting position.
- **Key points:** Keep the naval pulled in to protect the back.
- **Purpose:** To strengthen the outer thigh (abductors) and lateral flexors of the trunk.

STRETCHING EXERCISES

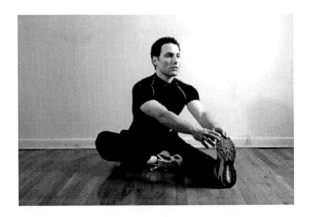

Knee to chest Stretch

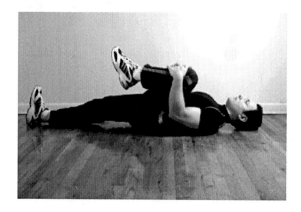

- **Action:** Lie down on your back and pull the knee into your chest. Hold for 15-30 seconds and repeat twice on each side.
- **Key points:** Keep the back flat against the floor.
- **Purpose:** To elongate the lower back and the gluteus maximus.

Curl Stretch

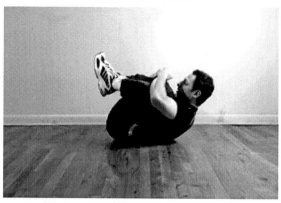

- **Action:** Lie down on your back and pull both knees into your chest. Place your face in between your knees. Hold for 15-30 seconds and repeat twice.
- **Key points:** Move into this position very fluidly. Never stretch if the pain is experienced.
- **Purpose:** To elongate the extensors of the spine.

Reclining Twist Stretch

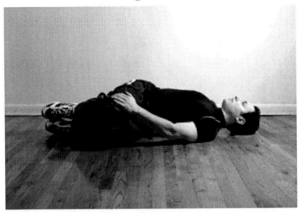

- **Action:** Lie down on your back. Bend the hips and knees in a 90 degree angle. Place both knees to the side on the ground. Hold for 15-30 seconds and repeat twice on each side.
- **Key points:** Keep the opposite shoulder on the floor.
- **Purpose:** To elongate the rotators of the trunk and gluteus.

Twisted Glute Stretch

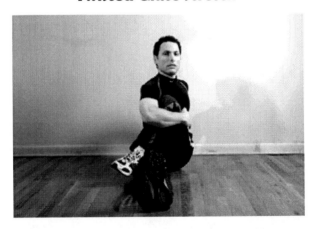

- **Action:** Have a seat with legs straight in front of you. Pull the inside of one knee into the opposite shoulder. Hold for 15-30 seconds and repeat twice on each side.
- **Key points:** Keep the trunk straight and vertical.
- **Purpose:** To elongate the gluteus and deep musculature of the hip joint.

Calve Stretch

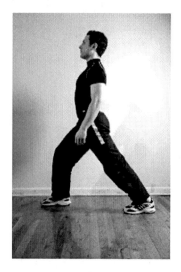

- **Action:** Stand with one foot in front of the other. Point the toes of both feet forward. Lean forward till the stretch is felt in the rear calf.
- **Key points:** Keep the rear heal on the floor. Make sure that both toes are pointed in the same direction.
- **Purpose:** To elongate the rear muscles of the lower leg.

Seated Hamstrings Stretch

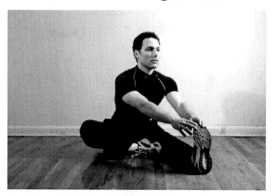

- **Action:** Have a seat on the floor and extend one leg forward Bend the other leg so that the foot of the bent leg is touching the inner thigh of the straight leg. Reach forward. Hold for 15-30 seconds and repeat twice on each side.
- **Key points:** Keep the back straight.
  Purpose: To elongate the hamstrings.

Mermaid Stretch

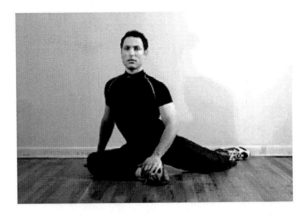

- **Action:** Sit with one leg bend in front and the other almost straight behind you. Keep extending the back leg till the stretch is felt. Hold for 15-30 seconds and repeat twice on each side.
- **Key points:** Keep the inside of the rear knee on the floor.
- **Purpose:** To lengthen the adductor muscles.

Quarter Split Stretch

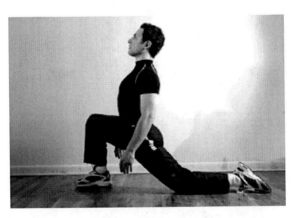

- **Action:** Place one leg flat on the ground so that the lower leg is vertical. Bring the other leg back as much as possible, so that the rear knee is behind the hip. Hold for 15-30 seconds and repeat twice on each side.
- **Key points:** Keep the rear knee cap pointing down.
- **Purpose:** To lengthen the hip flexors.

Cobra Stretch

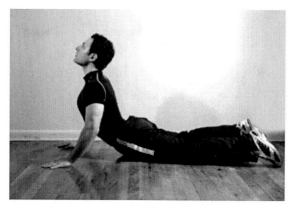

- **Action:** Lie down on your stomach, hands under the shoulders. Lift your head up, followed by the upper and middle back. Hold for 15-30 seconds and repeat twice.
- **Key points:** Keep the shoulders down and away from the ears. Do not bring the head all the way back.
- **Purpose:** To lengthen the abdominals.

Side Stretch

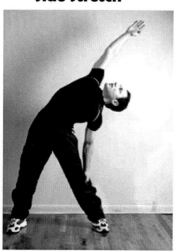

- **Action:** Stand with feet, shoulder width apart. Lean toward one side. Lift the opposite arm. Hold for 15-30 seconds and repeat twice on each side.
- **Key points:** Look up at your hand.
- **Purpose:** To stretch the major muscles located on the side of the body.

Posterior Deltoid Stretch

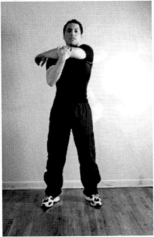

- **Action:** Place your left hand on the right shoulder. Place your right hand on the left elbow. Pull the left elbow across. Hold for 15-30 seconds and repeat twice on each side.
- **Key points:** Allow your shoulder blade to move naturally.
- **Purpose:** To elongate the muscles of the upper and middle back as well as the back of the shoulder.

Triceps Stretch

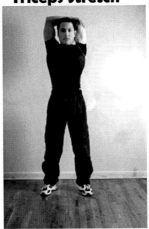

- **Action:** Bring your left elbow behind your head. With the right arms gently pull the elbow behind the head. Hold this position for 15-30 seconds, and repeat twice on each side.
- **Key points:** Do not allow the left elbow to press the head forward.
- **Purpose:** To loosen up the triceps, back of the shoulder, and shoulder adductors and extensors.

Upper Chest Opener

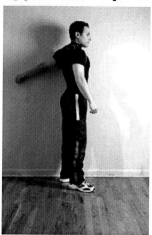

- **Action:** Stand side ways to the wall. Stretch the arm out and plac the palm on the wall. Rotate the body away from the wall till th stretch is felt. Hold for 15-30 seconds and repeat twice on each side
- **Key points:** Keep the hand below the shoulder.
- **Purpose:** To loosen up the muscles of the chest, anterior delto and biceps.

Lower Chest Opener

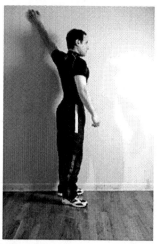

- **Action:** Stand sideway to the wall. Place one arm high on th wall. (Approximately 45 degrees up) Turn away from the wall, ti the stretch is felt. Hold for 15-30 seconds and repeat twice on eac side.
- **Key points:** Do not allow your lower back to arch.
- **Purpose:** To stretch the lower (sternal) part of the chest, as well a stabilizers of the shoulder girdle.

CROSS-REFERENCE

The cross reference index is designed for you to be able to pair up the muscle group and the exercise(s) that develop it.

There are six columns. The fist column gives the scientific name of the muscle group whose primary focus is to develop that muscle group. The second column lists the exercise who's primary focus is to develop that muscle group. For instance if the Deltoids is the muscle group, then Hand-Stand Press is one of the exercises, who's primary focus is to develop that muscle group.
Deltoids are the shoulders. You can see the translation in the fourth column. The third column is labeled "Secondary Use". This column lists the exercise, which develops the exercises listed in the corresponding row. However, the emphasis of these exercise on the corresponding muscle group is less than the ones listed in the second column. For instance dips work the shoulders, but their main focus is the chest.

The fourth column like stated above gives the common muscle name of the corresponding row. For instance, the adductors is the same thing as inner thigh.

Fifth row, lists the exercises that use the corresponding muscle groups as stabilizers. For instance the Glutes are the stabilizers for the Dragon Curl.

And finally, the last column lists the stretches. For instance the cobra is listed as the stretch for the abdominals.

Refer to this reference when you want to figure out how to develop or stretch a specific muscle group.

Cross-Reference		
Muscle Groups	**Primary Focus**	**Secondary Use**
Pectorals Major	Body Press Dips	Pull ups Hand Stand Press
Deltoid	Hand Stand Press Rocket	Dips Body Press Body Rows
Latissimus Dorsi	Body Rows Pull ups	N/A
Teres Major	Body Rows Pull ups	N/A
Trapezius	Handstand Press Rocket Body Rows Pull ups	N/A
Elbow Extensors	Body Press Hand Stand Press Dips	N/A
Elbow Flexors	Body Rows Rocket Pull ups	N/A
Wrist/Finger Flexors	N/A	N/A
Rectus Abdominis	N/A	Scissor planks
Obliques Abdominis	N/A	Scissor planks
Extensors of the Spine	N/A	Scissor planks
Gluteus Maximus	One leg squat Air Lunge	Open scissor plank
Hamstrings	Dragon Curl	Air Lunge
Quadriceps	Air Lunge One leg squat L-Extension Flag Extension	N/A
Hip Flexors	One leg squat	Air Lunge
Adductors	Scissors Close	Air Lunge One leg Squat
Abductors	Scissors Close	N/A
Calves	N/A	Air lunge Dragon Curl

Cross-Reference		
Muscle Groups	**Stabilization Use**	**Stretches**
Chest	N/A	Lower Chest Opener Upper Chest Opener
Shoulders	Pull ups	Upper Chest Opener Posterior Deltoid Stretch
Lats	Rocket	Side Stretch Triceps Stretch
Teres Major	Rocket	Side Stretch Triceps Stretch
Traps	Body Press	Posterior Deltoid Stretch
Triceps	Pull ups Body Rows Rocket	Triceps Stretch
Biceps	Body Press Hand Stand press	Upper Chest Opener (Palm must be facing down)
Hand/Finger Flexors	All Grip involving exercises	N/A
Abs	Most exercises	Cobra Side Stretch
Obliques	Most exercises	Cobra Side Stretch Reclining Glute Stretch
Back Muscles Parallel to Spine	Most exercises	One Knee Hug Curl Stretch Reclining Twist Side Stretch
Gluts	Dragon Curl	One Knee Hug Twisted Glute Stretch
Hamstrings	Scissor Planks One Leg Squats	Seated Hamstrings Strech
Quads	Scissor Planks	Quarter Split Stretch (Rear knee must be flexed and rear foot lifted.)
Front Upper Thigh	Most exercises	Quarter Split
Inner Thigh		Mermaid Stretch
Outer Thigh/Hip	Air Lunge One Leg Squat	Twisted Glute Stretch
Calves	One leg Squat Scissor Planks	Calve Stretch

OTHER BOOKS BY PAUL ZAICHIK

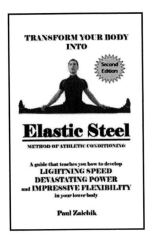

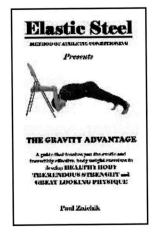

ElasticSteel Method of
Athletic Conditioning
Strength & Flexibility Book
$22.95

The Gravity Advantage
Upper Body Conditioning
$22.95

To order log on to www.ElasticSteel.com, www.GravityAdvantage.com, or fill out the order form below and send it to PMB 135, 7822 20th Avenue, Brooklyn, NY 11214. Make Check or Money Order payable to Paul Zaichik. Shipping & Handling Charges are $4.99 per book (USA) and $9.99 per book (Outside the US)

ORDER FORM

Item #	Description	Qty.	Price	Subtotal

Order total: _____

Method of Payment   ☐ Check   ☐ Money Order   ☐ Visa

Tax: _____

☐ MasterCard

Shipping: _____

Card # _____   Exp. date _____

☐ American Express

Total: _____

Signature